This Is NOT Normal!

A Busy Woman's Guide to Symptoms of Hormone Imbalance

This Is NOT Normal!

A Busy Woman's Guide to Symptoms of Hormone Imbalance

by Deborah Matthew, MD

ISBN: 978-1-945446-08-5

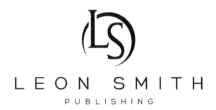

LEON SMITH
PUBLISHING

www.LeonSmithPublishing.com

Dedication

This book is dedicated to my husband, who taught me that anything is possible, but only if you are brave enough (or crazy enough) to try it.

Acknowledgments

I am indebted to the work of pioneering scientists and physicians who were brave enough to ask the questions that will lead to the rethinking of modern medicine. Instead of reflexive robotic diagnoses and treatment in five minutes or fewer, we need to return to intelligent contemplation of health issues as it relates to pharmaceuticals. My health, your health, and the future health of our families and this country depend on it.

I wish to thank Mark Houston, MD; Mark Hyman, MD; Patrick Hanaway, MD; Ron Rothenberg, MD; Philip Lee Miller, MD; Pam Smith, MD; Mehmet Oz, MD; Michael Roizen, MD; the American Academy of Anti-Aging and Regenerative Medicine; and the Institute for Functional Medicine, who have all given me new insight into healthcare.

I also wish to thank my husband and family for their love and support. I feel more fulfilled and educated now as a medical doctor. I feel a strong personal connection with my patients as I watch them get better after years and sometimes decades in which they did not feel normal.

Preface

You are a strong, capable woman.

Successful career? Check!

Friends and family? No problem!

A household that runs like a well-oiled machine? Well, sometimes at least.

Then, something happens to derail the train. You don't feel like yourself, and you just can't figure out why.

Do you have time to deal with this?

No way! Not with that presentation due at work tomorrow, the PTA meeting the next day, and twenty loads of laundry to do before the weekend. You get the picture.

Have you heard someone described as being "hormonal"?

Men think they're being funny when they say that, but there may be more truth to that phrase than we women care to believe.

Then along comes menopause. Whoa!

"What happens next?" you ask.

Many women look forward to life after menopause with foreboding, but it doesn't have to be that way. Additionally, menopause is not the only cause of hormone imbalances in women. Upon reading this book, you may be surprised by just how many things can cause hormone imbalances in women of all ages.

This book will be a huge asset to women navigating their life-long journey of wellness. I have presented critical information to you about symptoms of hormonal imbalances, their causes, and potential solutions.

We all know we have these things called *hormones* in our bodies.

However, where do they come from and what do they do?

You will be amazed to learn how complex the human hormone system really is! This book will demystify this complex system using clear, easy-to-understand language.

Each chapter will begin by presenting a case study. Hopefully, you will identify with the women in these stories and realize that these problems happen to real women, just like you. Then, each scenario will be explained in detail by describing what symptoms to look for in each hormonal imbalance and some of the mechanisms in your body that cause them. The pros and cons of various treatment options will also be discussed.

Each chapter also has a self-assessment quiz you can use to evaluate whether a condition applies to you. So, get out your number-two pencil, and get ready to learn more about yourself and have a little fun along the way.

Remember, there are symptoms that overlap in many conditions discussed in this book. These symptoms are also found in conditions not discussed in this book. So if you identify with a hormonal problem described here, make an appointment with your doctor. Armed with the information you have learned, you can talk to your healthcare provider more precisely about what you are experiencing. Then, working together, you can develop a plan that will restore you to the real you.

Be well!

Table of Contents

Introduction

Let's review the hormonal physiologic basics of what make women different than men. Women have a uterus and two ovaries. During puberty, women will experience their first period. A period occurs when the lining of the uterus, or the *endometrium*, is expelled from the body due to the absence of a fertilized egg.

There are hormonal changes that occur to promote endometrial thickening, the release of an egg, and the expulsion of endometrium. This is the menstrual cycle.

After the peak years of reproduction pass, the production of hormones start to decline. Estrogen, progesterone, and testosterone production start to fall. Eventually estrogen production becomes irregular. There may be times of excess or inadequate estrogen production. Sometimes there is a failure of ovulation and this results in a lack of progesterone production. These are signs of pre-exhaustion of the ovaries, also called *perimenopause*. Decline in a hormone may start up to ten years before menopausal symptoms are noticeable.

These irregularities are associated with all the symptoms that typically occur in perimenopause. These symptoms can be teased out and attributed to inadequate levels of estrogen, progesterone, or testosterone. This is discussed further in later chapters.

Perimenopause can be one of the most difficult transitions in a women's life. Sadly, some women are told to tough it out and that it will pass. While it is true that the wide fluctuations in hormone levels and their associated symptom roller coaster will come to an end, the damage is just starting.

Deficiencies in these hormones contribute to some of the biggest health issues that face postmenopausal women today. These issues include osteoporosis, bone fractures, dementia, heart disease, mood changes, and more.

Hormone balancing is not a cure-all, and my intent is not to portray it as such. However, it is an often-overlooked area that has important implications for every woman's current and future health.

Chapter One

What's Wrong Here?

You have successfully dropped two of your three children at the bus stop, cleared the breakfast dishes, cleaned a blob of oatmeal off your silk blouse, handed off a dry cleaning ticket to your husband with a quick kiss, dropped off the three-year-old at daycare, and you are now sitting at a red light on your way to work. Your cell phone rings. A client is calling to reschedule a meeting for later this afternoon.

With a heavy sigh, you speed-dial your husband to see if he is available to pick up your youngest at daycare.

Suddenly, you think: *I used to thrive on the adrenaline rush of successfully juggling family and career. What happened? I don't think I have the energy to get to work, let alone make it through the rest of the day. What's wrong here?*

You may just be tired.

No, that's not it. You feel like something has changed. You don't feel *normal* anymore.

You may be like numerous successful women who are used to performing at a high level and then one day slam headlong into an invisible roadblock. Your energy is gone. You become forgetful, irritable, and overly emotional — you're no longer on your game.

There is hope!

In this book you will answer a few questions and read several scenarios of women who may have symptoms similar to yours. If any of the scenarios ring true for you, you have taken the first step in identifying symptoms of hormonal imbalance that can be treated in a number of ways.

This book is not meant to be a cure on its own. It will provide you with information about symptoms of hormonal imbalance and possible treatments. Once you are armed with the valuable information contained in these pages, you may decide to speak with your doctor or make simple changes in your lifestyle to see if they produce positive results.

So, take a few minutes, relax, and see if you find yourself in these pages.

There are solutions.

You are not alone.

You can feel normal again!

Chapter Two

I Didn't Know
There Would Be a Test

Don't worry. You know the answers to this test — it's all about you.

First, let's start with a little background information. Each woman's hormonal makeup is unique. There is no one exact hormonal recipe for the perfectly healthy woman — one half-cup of estrogen, a pinch of testosterone, and so on. It just doesn't work that way. Your hormonal balance is as individual as you are.

Every hormone in your body affects every other hormone. So, if the amount of estrogen you are producing starts to change, for example, there is a domino effect that reaches every other hormone in your system. Hormones do not work independently. They are intertwined in a beautiful tapestry that is uniquely yours.

Further, there is no way to pinpoint exactly when your hormonal balance may change. The normal age for menopause is not very exact. Menopause can begin anywhere from age thirty-five through fifty-five. Things like stress, changes in diet, and lack of exercise can also affect your hormonal balance.

The good news is that experts have identified signs of hormonal changes, and we can now often pinpoint exactly which hormone is out of balance, depending on the nature of your symptoms.

Let's start with a short, general quiz, just to get you thinking about how you are feeling from the inside out.

Please rate each of the following symptoms on a scale of 0 to 3:

0 = Does not apply to me
1 = Maybe a little bit
2 = Happens often
3 = All the time

_3_ Fatigue

_1_ Anxiety

_2_ Irritability

_1_ Difficulty coping with stress

_1_ Depression

_1_ Cry easily

_1_ Major mood swings

_2_ Sleepy during the day

_2_ Forgetful

_0_ Headaches/Migraines

_3_ Cold hands and feet

_2_ Dizzy or lightheadedness

_2_ Dry skin

_1_ Hair falling out

_3_ Brittle nails

_2_ Craving sweet or salty foods

_3_ Bloating

_3_ Weight gain

_1_ Tender breasts

_3_ Vaginal dryness

_1_ Not interested in sex anymore

_2_ Insomnia

_6_ Wake up hot at night

_6_ Sweat easily or at unexpected times

What is your total score? _40_

If your total score is less than seven, hormone imbalance may not be an issue for you. It might be time to explore other reasons with your physician for why you don't feel quite normal. Feel free to keep reading, though. A particular chapter in this book may still ring true for you and provide you with a clue to this complicated puzzle we call the human body.

If your total score is between seven and eleven, you may be able to correct occasional symptoms of hormonal imbalance easily through natural changes that will be detailed later in this book.

If your total score is more than twelve, it is likely that you have a hormonal imbalance that needs attention. You may want to look into ways you can improve your overall health and correct some of these imbalances. This book will be a great start for you, as well as talking with your physician about options.

Now, let's break down some of these symptoms. The following chapters will look at the most common hormone imbalances in women.

Chapter Three

Getting on My Last Nerve—
Progesterone Deficiency

Anne was on the phone catching up with her college roommate. After a few rounds of the Ohio State fight song and fits of giggles, they got down to more serious topics.

"I am lucky to have a good-natured husband, because lately things have been getting difficult," Anne confided. "Some days I still feel like the fun-loving, energetic girl he married and other days I snap at him and the kids and it seems like everything is just so incredibly irritating!"

"Don't we all have days like that?"

"But this is out of control. Some days even I don't like myself! This can't be normal!"

Anne recognized that this was more than a few bad days. Her husband saw the changes too. He had taken to calling her on the way home from work—he could tell by the way she answered the phone whether this was a good day or whether he would need to tread softly.

Anne was concerned—she didn't understand where these mood swings were coming from. She knew she wasn't sleeping as well and that wasn't helping. But some days every little thing just got on her last nerve and she felt a little crazy.

* * *

Anne probably isn't going crazy. She may be suffering from progesterone deficiency.

There are a number of causes of low progesterone, and we will go over them in this chapter.

First, let's go over some additional hormonal basics.

Progesterone is produced in two main places in the female body. It is produced in the ovaries and in the adrenal glands. The majority of progesterone in women is produced in the ovaries after ovulation. It helps to prepare the uterine lining in case of a pregnancy and is very important throughout pregnancy (it is "progestational").

When a woman is in the second half of her monthly cycle, she is producing between twenty and twenty-five milligrams of progesterone a day. During pregnancy, production of progesterone spikes to between 300 and 400 milligrams per day.

After menopause, a woman's production of progesterone drops dramatically. It can end up at less than 1 percent of what it was before menopause.

Progesterone is extremely important to hormonal synthesis. It is used to make estrogen, testosterone, and cortisol. So progesterone is an important link in the hormonal balance of your body.

While estrogen levels start to decline around the time of menopause, progesterone levels start to decline much earlier. In fact, a woman's progesterone production may decline by as much as 80 percent between ages thirty and forty. This is one of the reasons women in their forties have a harder time getting pregnant.

When progesterone levels start to decline because of age, and symptoms of hormone imbalance become noticeable, we call this *perimenopause.*

Progesterone deficiency is the most common hormonal problem we see in perimenopausal women, but younger women can also have this problem. Because progesterone levels naturally vary over the menstrual cycle, the symptoms vary as well.

Typically the week after a period is a good week; you are eating your broccoli, exercising regularly, and cleaning out your closets. As you get closer to your period, symptoms get worse and worse, including irritability, anxiousness, and interrupted sleep. You may feel more negative, critical, impatient, and easily frustrated—and this can affect how you behave toward your family and co-workers.

In fact, this variation in symptoms is a big clue that hormones are the problem. If your mood symptoms or insomnia are exactly the same on every day in your cycle, it is less likely that hormones are the cause.

Progesterone has been studied mainly for its effects on the uterus, but it turns out that progesterone has far more roles to play. Women have progesterone receptors on cells in all parts of our bodies, and surprisingly the cells with the most progesterone receptors are our brain cells. Anyone who has experienced PMS symptoms with mood swings and irritability may not be surprised after all.

Research is showing that progesterone has important neurological effects. It acts as a natural anti-anxiety compound, helps with sleep and is calming—sort of like nature's version of Valium or a glass of red wine.

Estrogen and progesterone are in sync because they are opposites. In other words, they have opposing effects on your body.

Here are a few examples of the ways in which estrogen and progesterone affect both sides of the seesaw, so that your body remains in perfect balance:

- Estrogen increases salt and water retention, while progesterone is a natural diuretic.

- Estrogen may promote cysts in your breast tissue. Progesterone protects against breast cysts.

- Some types of estrogen have been associated with promoting breast and endometrial cancer. Progesterone protects against cancer.

- Estrogen stimulates growth of the uterine lining, while progesterone inhibits growth and causes the lining to mature. An imbalance may result in heavy, frequent, or irregular periods.

- Estrogen is energizing to the brain and progesterone has calming effects. An imbalance may result in anxiety or irritability.

Let's take the quiz.

Answer YES or NO to the following questions:

Do you have insomnia or trouble sleeping?	(YES)	NO
Do you have painful or lumpy breasts?	YES	(NO)
Do you have heavy bleeding or clots during your period?	(YES)	NO

Do you have irregular periods? (YES) NO

Do your periods come more frequently
    than twenty-eight days apart? YES (NO)

Do you have major mood swings? YES (NO)

Do you have night sweats? YES (NO)

Do you suffer from PMS? YES (NO)

Do you get headaches associated
    with your period? YES (NO)

Have you experienced infertility? YES (NO)

Have you recently had an unexplained
    weight gain? (YES) NO

Have you had an early miscarriage? YES (NO)

Do you tend to be anxious? YES (NO)

Are you more irritable or impatient
    than in the past? (YES) NO

If you answered YES to fewer than five of the questions above, low progesterone is not likely to be an issue for you.

If you answered YES to between five and seven of the questions above, you may have a progesterone deficiency.

If you answered YES to eight or more questions above, it is likely that your progesterone levels are low.

If you answered YES to a lot of the questions on this quiz, you are not alone. Progesterone deficiency is the most common hormonal imbalance in women, regardless of age.

Progesterone has many functions in the body:

- It acts as a diuretic.
- It protects the uterus, breasts, and ovaries from cancer.
- It reduces anxiety.
- It helps form new bone tissue.
- It helps support thyroid and adrenal function.
- It helps promote deep, restorative sleep.

When women experience progesterone loss, not only are the above functions in jeopardy, but the entire hormonal balance can easily be affected. Take a close look at the symptoms of progesterone deficiency to see if many of these symptoms describe you.

Here is a more complete list of symptoms and signs of progesterone deficiency:

- Mood swings
- Heavy/excessive menstruation
- More frequent periods (cycles last fewer than twenty-eight days)
- Irregular cycles
- Irritability
- Depression
- Pre-menstrual headaches
- Anxiety
- Tender breasts
- Strong symptoms of PMS
- Infertility
- Insomnia (waking at night)
- Fluid retention
- Bloating
- Loss of libido

- Fibroids
- Ovarian cysts
- Night sweats
- Sweet cravings
- Weight gain
- Mood swings
- Fibrocystic or lumpy breasts

Another symptom that tends to go hand in hand with progesterone deficiency is low thyroid function. Progesterone gives aid to the thyroid gland, so if progesterone is low, chances are thyroid function may not be optimal.

Keep in mind that progesterone and estrogen have opposing actions in the body. So, excess estrogen or insufficient progesterone both result in what we call *estrogen dominance* and cause similar symptoms.

See what a domino effect these hormones have on each other?

They are certainly intertwined.

Other than perimenopause, what might cause low progesterone levels?

Diet could be one of the culprits. A diet high in sugar and saturated fat can throw off your body's production of progesterone.

Also, a deficiency in the following vitamins and minerals can lower progesterone levels:

- Vitamin A
- Vitamin B6
- Vitamin C
- Zinc
- Magnesium

Over the last hundred years or so, the diet of an average woman in the United States has moved away from whole foods (fruits and vegetables in particular) to more processed food. These modern conveniences are inundating the system with estrogen-like environmental chemicals that may be throwing your hormonal systems off balance.

In addition, decreased thyroid hormone could result in lower progesterone levels. A common complaint in women with hypothyroidism (underfunctioning thyroid gland) is menstrual irregularities with heavy periods. Sound familiar?

Another common reason for low progesterone levels is excess stress. As your stress levels increase, your body produces more of the stress hormone *cortisol* at the expense of progesterone.

Many women find that when they are under significant stress their PMS symptoms or menopausal symptoms are worse, and as the stress levels decrease their symptoms also calm down.

If you are under a lot of stress, your levels of progesterone may be lower than usual and dealing with the underlying problem (stress!) may help. This is covered in an upcoming chapter.

Have you determined that you may be suffering from progesterone deficiency?

Experienced physicians in the area of bioidentical hormone replacement therapy can offer testing that will measure hormone levels in your body and, more important, know how to interpret the results. There is an art to it. Find an experienced physician or the results may be disappointing.

If you decide be tested, it is important that you take the test on a day when your symptoms are strong, typically about one week before your period is due. Then, you can get an accurate reading of your hormone levels when you are feeling particularly NOT normal.

There are many testing options available, including blood, urine, and saliva testing. Your physician can recommend a lab. There are certain standards of testing that make some labs better than others. There are also certain circumstances where a healthcare provider may prefer one type of test to another.

Often saliva tests are a good option when looking for progesterone deficiency in premenopausal women, because the saliva test labs are set up to look for optimal progesterone levels — levels where women are less likely to have hormonal symptoms. Blood tests are set up to look for serious diseases, like tumors, and are sometimes less helpful.

If testing shows that you are low in progesterone, there are a number of ways in which you can try to increase your level.

First, you can change your diet to include whole, unprocessed foods and cut down your consumption of sugar and starchy carbohydrates. Add ground flaxseeds and healthy fats to your diet, including fish, nuts, and avocado. You can also try supplementing with Vitamins A, B6, C, and zinc.

Another option is to add natural, bioidentical progesterone.

Natural, Bioidentical Progesterone

In this context, the word bioidentical means that the progesterone molecule used is an exact match to what your ovaries make. So in theory, your body should not be able to tell whether the progesterone came from your ovaries or the pharmacy.

Natural progesterone has a number of positive effects in the body:

- ☐ Balances estrogen

- ☐ Improves sleep

- ☐ Lowers cholesterol

- ☐ Leaves the body quickly

- ☐ Naturally calms you, even sometimes lowering high blood pressure

- ☐ Aids the body in using and eliminating fats

- ☐ Natural antidepressant

- ☐ Natural diuretic

- ☐ May protect against uterine and breast cancer

- ☐ Increases healthy scalp hair

- ☐ Increases metabolism

Literature supporting favorable effects on cardiovascular function is growing.

Natural, bioidentical progesterone has been used for more than thirty years and is available as an FDA-approved capsule or in compounded formulations (topical or vaginal creams, capsules, or sublingual troches). Once your symptoms are confirmed and hormone levels are measured, your doctor can formulate a dosage to restore normal hormonal balance.

For some women, taking progesterone as a pill may be a better option. The pill form of progesterone may help more with anxiety, irritability, and insomnia.

On the other hand, the cream form is preferred for some women who feel *too* sleepy on progesterone pills.

Caution must be used in premenopausal women taking progesterone, as it may *increase* fertility (after all it is *pro-gestational!*)

Synthetic Progestins

Synthetic progesterone medications are called *progestins* or *progestagens*. These are chemicals that have been manufactured to mimic the functions of progesterone, but the molecule is *not* exactly the same. Therefore the effects are not exactly the same.

Synthetic progestins are used in birth control pills. They may also be used in menopausal hormone replacement therapy.

There are many different types of progestin medications, and they are sometimes suggested as a means to increase the level of progesterone in your body. It is important to know that they do not behave in the body in quite the same way as the natural progesterone your body produces.

The words *progestin* and *progesterone* are often used interchangeably even though they are clearly different:

Synthetic progestins and natural progesterone are NOT the same. *The effects of progestins on the uterus are the same as the effects of natural progesterone, but outside the uterus the effects are different, and often the opposite.*

The side effects of progestin drugs are often the same as the symptoms of low progesterone. In general, if you read about progesterone in the media, it is likely that they are talking about synthetic progestins. Many doctors are not aware that there is any difference.

There is a long list of side effects associated with progestins.

Here are just a few of the known side effects:

- Increase in appetite
- Depression
- Bloating
- Tender breasts
- Irritability
- Headaches
- Acne
- Hair loss
- Nausea

Additionally, progestins remain in the body longer than natural hormones. They block some of the heart protection provided by estrogen. This may partly explain the **higher rate of heart attacks** and strokes in women taking *medroxyprogesterone acetate* or MPA, the most common progestin used in synthetic hormone replacement therapy for menopausal women.

One final reason that progestins may not be a great option is that they may make the symptoms of progesterone deficiency even worse. **Progestins interfere with your body's production of natural progesterone**.

As you can see, many of the side effects are the very symptoms you are trying to get rid of in the first place. Synthetic progestins may be something you want to avoid.

So, why take a progestin? Exactly!

What about postmenopausal women? Do they need progesterone too?

Many menopausal women who are on hormone replacement with estrogen alone are not happy with the results. They are gaining weight in their hips and abdomen; they have little or no sex drive; and on top of that, their breasts feel tender and swollen.

Progesterone is needed, as well as testosterone, to make sure that the desired ratio remains the same in your body. When you double a recipe, you have to adjust all the ingredients, not just one.

An example of this interaction is demonstrated by the fact that natural progesterone is actually required for the optimal functioning of estrogen. Even if the estrogen dose remains unchanged, adding progesterone (or switching from a synthetic progestin to natural progesterone) may result in an increase in estrogen function.

Traditionally, progesterone has been used in women on menopausal estrogen replacement who have their uterus (but not in women who have had a hysterectomy). Estrogen replacement can stimulate the growth of the uterine lining and increase the risk of uterine cancer. Progesterone prevents this risk.

Unfortunately, there is an increased risk of breast cancer with the use of synthetic progestins. For this reason, your doctor may not offer you progestin treatment if you have had a hysterectomy. You don't have to worry about uterine cancer, so why would you want to increase your risk of breast cancer, or worry about the side effects of progestin treatment?

Studies show that natural, bioidentical progesterone does not increase the risk of breast cancer.

Natural progesterone has many beneficial effects on other parts of the body, including brain, bones, thyroid, and adrenals. Even a woman without a uterus can benefit from progesterone replacement.

It promotes improved quality of sleep, calm mood, and is a feel-good hormone. These are all very important for quality of life.

So you have decided to start on bioidentical progesterone treatment. What next?

Periodic hormone tests are typically done to check your hormonal levels and assess changes. Not all doctors are familiar or experienced in adjusting progesterone. Remember, your hormone balance is a delicate, interwoven tapestry that is unique to you. Altering one hormone may alter another.

Make sure your physician has experience in this area. If your doctor thinks that progestin is the same as progesterone, then you have your answer — they do not have experience.

The key point here is that you want to maintain a certain ratio of progesterone to estrogen to obtain the maximum benefits.

If you use natural progesterone cream or capsules for a prolonged period of time, but you do not have adequate estrogen levels in your system, the following could result:

- Increase in triglycerides (fats found in the bloodstream)
- Increase in feelings of depression
- Increase in insulin resistance
- Decrease in libido
- Increase in LDL ("bad" cholesterol)
- Decrease in HDL ("good" cholesterol)

- Increase in weight
- Increase in fatigue

If you decide to take natural progesterone hormones, it is very important to remember that a little dab will do the trick. Women often respond to low doses of progesterone. More is not always better.

It is very rare to have excess levels of progesterone naturally; excess progesterone is usually due to an excessive dose of progesterone replacement.

Symptoms that may be seen with too much progesterone replacement include:

- Heartburn
- Weight gain
- Insulin resistance (requires a blood test to diagnose)
- Drowsiness
- Depressed feeling
- Slight dizziness
- Increased breast tenderness
- Waking up groggy
- Heaviness of the extremities
- Decreased libido
- Increased water retention

If these symptoms seem to describe you to a T, and you are currently using progesterone replacement, you may want to discontinue use and see if the symptoms cease. Let your progesterone level drop a little, so that it is back within a normal range for you.

There are a small number of women who simply do not tolerate progesterone pills due to side effects. A topical form may work much better.

An even smaller group of women also do not tolerate the cream. You may be one of these women, and that could also be the reason for your symptoms. Speak with your doctor about the possibility of having intolerance to progesterone.

Human beings may be 99 percent the same, but that pesky 1 percent makes each of us unique. You have a distinctive hormonal ratio that is yours alone, so you may have to do a little trial and error to find out what works and what does not. More importantly, you need a healthcare provider who is willing to spend the time to work with you and find your unique formula.

Chapter Four

Too Much of a Good Thing—
Estrogen Excess

Jean is thirty-five years old. She is a marketing executive on the fast track to success. She is happily married, and she and her husband, Bill, are considering having children. Jean makes an appointment to visit her OB/GYN to talk with her about prenatal vitamins. She also takes this opportunity to speak with her doctor about some recent symptoms that are causing concern.

Jean has been having a lot of trouble sleeping lately. She does not believe her insomnia is due to stress at work, because nothing much has changed on the job in the last few months. In fact, she usually thrives on stress and enjoys the fast pace and excitement of her career. However, lately she has noticed that she is more irritable than usual at the office and with her husband of five years.

Jean's doctor asks a few follow-up questions and discovers that Jean is also having unusually heavy periods, and her breasts seem to be very swollen and tender right before her period. In addition, Jean has gained about ten pounds since her last checkup.

Jean's doctor begins to consider the fact that Jean may be exhibiting the signs of estrogen excess.

* * *

One of the primary roles of estrogen is to regulate a woman's reproductive system. However, estrogen affects quite a few other areas of the body, from the purely physical to the emotional. You may be surprised to note that estrogen actually has over four hundred functions in the body.

Here are a few of the things that estrogen can do:

- ☐ Increases metabolism
- ☐ Prevents Alzheimer's disease
- ☐ Improves sleep
- ☐ Maintains muscle tissue
- ☐ Regulates body temperature
- ☐ Increases blood flow
- ☐ Reduces risk of cataracts
- ☐ Helps with fine motor skills
- ☐ Increases water content of skin
- ☐ Increases ability to reason
- ☐ Maintains bone density
- ☐ Improves mood
- ☐ Increases energy
- ☐ Reduces risk of heart disease

- ☐ Increases sexual interest

- ☐ Decreases risk of colon cancer

- ☐ Decreases blood pressure

- ☐ Maintains memory

You certainly would like to have all of the above in abundance. So, bring it on, right? Actually, too much estrogen can be a little like too much chocolate: There is eventually a bad side.

It's time for another quiz!

Circle YES or NO in response to the following questions:

Do you feel bloated before your period?	YES	NO
Are your breasts tender before your period?	YES	NO
Do you have mood swings?	YES	NO
Do you get frequent headaches or migraines?	YES	NO
Do you have endometriosis?	YES	NO
Do you suffer from anxiety?	YES	NO
Have you recently gained a significant amount of weight?	YES	NO
Do you have uterine fibroids?	YES	NO
Are your cycles less than twenty-eight days?	YES	NO
Are your periods heavy?	YES	NO
Do you have fibrocystic breasts?	YES	NO
Have you noticed a decrease in your libido?	YES	NO

Do you have premenstrual water retention
    and weight gain?   YES   NO

Now count the number of times you answered YES to the questions above.

Total number of yes answers: _____

If you answered YES to five or fewer questions, you probably do not have excess estrogen.

If you answered YES to between six and ten questions, it is possible that estrogen excess is an issue for you.

If you answered YES to more than ten questions, it is probable that excess estrogen exists in your system.

Having your hormone levels tested can confirm the problem.

You may have noticed that the symptoms of estrogen excess and the symptoms of progesterone deficiency are very similar. Both result in *estrogen dominance*, meaning that there is a loss of balance between the effects of estrogen and effects of progesterone — the see-saw of hormonal balance is tipped too far in the estrogen direction.

A lab test may be necessary to determine whether the problems are due to low progesterone or too much estrogen.

There are a number of reasons why you may have excess estrogen in your body. One reason may be that you are taking too much estrogen, either through an oral contraceptive or a hormone replacement that is meant to offset the symptoms of menopause.

Here are some other possible causes of high estrogen:

- Ovarian cysts or tumors, which cause an overproduction of estrogen. Fortunately, this is rare.

- Liver disease, which limits the breakdown of estrogen, allowing levels to accumulate.

- Obesity. Body fat cells make estrogen. In an obese individual, excess production of estrogen may result.

- High blood sugar triggers the enzyme that generates estrogen in body fat tissues.

- Increase in caffeine consumption. Studies have shown that women who drink four to five cups of coffee a day have almost 70 percent more estrogen than women who drink only one cup a day.

- Drinking an excessive amount of alcohol. Even as few as two drinks a day can impair liver function enough to reduce estrogen clearance and elevate estrogen levels in women.

Excess estrogen may also be a result of something as simple as lack of exercise or a diet that is low in fiber.

Here is a more comprehensive list of symptoms and conditions associated with estrogen excess:

- Bloating
- Water retention
- Fatigue
- Swollen breasts
- Headaches
- Insomnia

- Uterine fibroids
- Hypothyroidism
- Irritability
- Mood swings
- Food cravings
- Migraines
- Anxiety
- Endometriosis
- Fibrocystic breasts
- Increased risk for breast cancer
- Depression
- Heavy periods
- Anxiety
- Weight gain (particularly in abdomen, hips, and thighs)
- Mood swings
- Hair loss
- Gallbladder pain from gallstones

If your symptoms are not severe, there are many steps you can take on your own to naturally offset estrogen excess. Eating cruciferous vegetables and adding ground flaxseed to your diet may help reverse the effects of an excess of estrogen.

Here are a few additional suggestions to naturally decrease the estrogen in your system:

- Decrease the saturated and trans fat in your diet.

- Decrease sugar in your diet.

- Decrease grains and pasta in your diet.

- Increase high-fiber foods in your diet, such as vegetables, particularly cruciferous vegetables (e.g., cauliflower, broccoli, cabbage, Brussels sprouts, kale).

- Increase healthy proteins in your diet (like organic, lean meat and wild-caught fish.)

- Take B6 supplements (pyridoxine-5-phosphate is the activated form of B6).

- Try chasteberry supplements (also called *vitex*).

- Include 2 tablespoons/day of ground flaxseed in your diet (add to smoothies or mix into your food).

- Increase your exercise regimen. Try to get in at least four 30-minute sessions of brisk activity per week.

- Lower your consumption of alcohol.

- Take milk thistle (also called *silymarin*) to support liver function.

- Look for organic milk and cheese.

- Add natural progesterone to balance the effects of estrogen.

You could also speak with your healthcare provider about discontinuing the use of an oral contraceptive or adjusting the dose of your estrogen hormone replacement, if you are currently taking either of those.

The Environment Can Also Play a Role in the Amount of Estrogen in Your System.

Xenoestrogens are chemicals in the environment that act like estrogen. They are known as *endocrine disruptors*. It is likely that xenoestrogens could be part of the cause of an epidemic of female diseases that are traceable to excess estrogen.

There are approximately fifty chemicals that imitate estrogen and can be toxic to your body. They are found in:

- Pesticide residues in your food
- Parabens found in cosmetics, creams, lotions, shampoos
- Plastics (phthalates and bis-phenol A or BPA)
- Synthetic hormones that are fed to animals

Well, what can you do about that?

Actually, there are some things you *can* do:

- Pay close attention to your diet, and try to eat organic foods whenever possible to decrease your exposure to xenoestrogens.

- Buy organic milk and butter as a priority (many dairy cows are treated with hormones).

- Wash your food well.

- Check the labels of your beauty products and look for the word "parabens".

- Throw out anything that contains parabens.

- Don't microwave in plastic. Use glass containers instead.

- Minimize your use of plastic water bottles. The phthalates leach out more when the plastic is heated or cooled.

- Avoid canned foods because the lining of the can contains BPA.

You may not be able to completely remove yourself from xenoestrogens in the environment, but you can certainly lower your exposure by taking a look at ingredients in the food you eat and the cosmetics you wear.

Chapter Five

Feeling HOT But Not Sexy—
Estrogen Deficiency

Cindy is forty-eight years old. She owns a thriving arts and crafts business, and by most accounts, her life is moving along fabulously. She meets a friend for lunch and shares a laugh about how she seems to be flipping out these days.

"Maybe it's early stages of Alzheimer's — or maybe I should call it half-zheimer's! I'm halfway to the grave!" She giggles, but she's only half joking.

Cindy has stopped counting the number of times she walks into a room in her home and forgets why she's there. She's thinking about attaching her keys and her glasses to her body at all times. Her husband found her opening windows in her craft studio and hanging her head out the window to cool off — it was February in northern Minnesota! Hot flashes are not for sissies, she informs her friend.

* * *

If forgetfulness is something that you are suffering from as well, you are not alone. Changes in speech, memory, and behavior are very common complaints of women going through menopause. Estrogen deficiency is one of the reasons for these changes.

Here are a few common observations of women who have experienced changes in speech, memory, and behavior during menopause:

- Word retrieval, or not being able to find the right word. Relying on "what's his name" or "whatchamacallit" to fill in for gaps in recall.

- Feeling foggy or like there is cotton in your head, and having a hard time shaking the feeling and getting clear.

- Unable to prioritize tasks as easily as you have in the past.

- Briefly forgetting how to do things you do all the time, like setting your house alarm.

- Not handling stress as well as you used to.

Test time again! Please take this short quiz to see if you may be suffering from estrogen deficiency.

Circle YES or NO in response to the following questions:

Are your periods becoming very light and infrequent?	YES	NO
Have your periods ended?	YES	NO
Do you feel more tired?	YES	NO
Are you having memory problems?	YES	NO
Have you gained weight?	YES	NO
Do you suffer with dry eyes?	YES	NO
Do you have problems finding the word you want?	YES	NO

Do you have a hard time falling asleep?	YES	NO
Do you randomly break out in a sweat?	YES	NO
Are you depressed?	YES	NO
Have you lost interest in sex?	YES	NO
Do you have vaginal dryness?	YES	NO
Do you urinate frequently?	YES	NO
Do you often feel like your heart is racing?	YES	NO
Have you noticed an increase in facial hair?	YES	NO
Is your skin dry or itchy?	YES	NO

Add up the number of times you answered YES to the questions above.

Total number of YES answers: _____

If you have answered YES to fewer than five questions, you probably do not suffer from estrogen deficiency.

If you answered YES to between five and seven questions, you may have some estrogen deficiency.

If you answered YES to eight or more questions, it is likely that you are suffering from estrogen deficiency.

Remember that estrogen has more than four hundred functions in the body. It is one powerful hormone! Here are a few of the amazing things that estrogen can do:

- Increases metabolism
- Prevents Alzheimer's disease
- Improves sleep

- Maintains muscle tissue
- Regulates body temperature
- Increases blood flow
- Reduces risk of cataracts
- Helps with fine motor skills
- Increases water content of skin
- Increases ability to reason
- Maintains bone density
- Improves mood
- Increases energy
- Reduces risk of heart disease
- Increases sexual interest
- Decreases risk of colon cancer
- Decreases blood pressure
- Maintains memory

Irregular or missed periods are some of the main symptoms of estrogen deficiency, and they can occur not just in menopause, but also in the years leading up to menopause. This also happens in women whose ovaries have been damaged or surgically removed, regardless of age.

A woman is said to be menopausal when she has gone for one full year without a period. The average age is fifty-two, but there is a great deal of variation. The period of time leading up to menopause is called *perimenopause*, and the symptoms of perimenopause may last for many years.

The most visible signals of estrogen deficiency are changes in skin health. The skin bruises more easily and becomes dry, itchy, and less elastic. Plus, your skin may become thinner and more wrinkled, due to decreased levels of collagen.

Osteoporosis (thin, fragile bones) has also been linked to estrogen deficiency. Lack of calcium, vitamin D, and vitamin K may also be involved.

Vaginal dryness is another common symptom of estrogen deficiency, and it may cause painful intercourse, which leads to decreased sex drive in women.

Weight gain is unfortunately common as well. The average woman gains twenty pounds as she goes through menopause.

Here are a few signs and symptoms of estrogen deficiency:

- Bloating
- Recent weight gain
- Low back pain
- Poor memory
- Rapid pulse or palpitations
- Vaginal dryness
- Hot flashes
- Lethargy and fatigue
- Osteoporosis or osteopenia
- Decreased sex drive
- Bladder control issues/frequent urination
- Dry, itchy skin
- Depression
- Headaches
- Joint pain or stiffness
- Dry mouth
- Dry eyes

Now you may be thinking: *Bingo! I've got this one. Tell me what I can do to make these things go away.*

Let's go over a few tips you can do right now to help alleviate some of the symptoms.

- Exercise more. Try to get in at least four 30-minute sessions of brisk activity per week.

- Increase your general activity. Take the stairs instead of the elevator; park at the other end of the parking lot so you are forced to walk farther; play with your kids more; take a walk with your significant other in the evening or early morning.

- Eat healthier. Reexamine your diet and make healthy changes, which include more organic foods.

- Lower your stress whenever possible.

Estrogen Replacement: Is It Safe?

Currently estrogen replacement is FDA approved for the treatment of hot flashes and night sweats and for protection from osteoporosis. It also decreases the incidence of colon cancer.

Research is showing that starting estrogen replacement early (at the time of menopause) may help prevent Alzheimer's disease and heart disease, and more studies continue to look at these issues.

So why are many women fearful of taking estrogen?

Women's Health Initiative Study

The preliminary results of the *Women's Health Initiative Trial* were published in 2002, and they certainly got a lot of attention.

Many physicians were concerned and decided to avoid prescribing hormone replacement therapy.

Many women became nervous about taking hormones after hearing about this study, and overall, hormone replacement got a bad rap. But let's take a closer look.

In this study, women were given a pill with conjugated equine estrogen (CEE, which is a combination of estrogens derived from horse urine), and medroxy progesterone acetate (MPA, a chemical that mimics progesterone). At the time of the study, this pill was the most standard form of hormone replacement used.

The study results showed that out of ten thousand women taking this pill, there were seven more heart attacks, eight more blood clots in the lungs, eight more strokes, and eight more instances of breast cancer compared with women given a placebo pill. Not insignificant numbers.

On the other hand, there were six fewer instances of colorectal cancer and five fewer hip fractures. Based on these results, the media widely spread the word that hormone replacement therapy causes breast cancer.

The WHI study is misleading. Why?

1. The hormones used were not bioidentical. Human women do not have CEE or MPA in their bodies. CEE is metabolized differently than the estrogen that women make in their ovaries. MPA is classified by the World Health Organization (WHO) as a known carcinogen. On the other hand, progesterone (the kind made in a woman's ovaries) has not been shown in clinical studies to increase the risk of breast cancer.

2. Oral hormones were used. When estrogen is swallowed, it can be transformed into dangerous byproducts as it passes through the liver after being absorbed from the gut. This results in an increased production of blood clotting factors and inflammatory proteins (both of which are implicated in the risk for strokes and heart attacks).

When estrogen is given by an alternate route, such as topically through the skin, it does not pass through the liver, and we do not see an increase in blood clots.

3. The women in the study were older. The average age of women in the study was sixty-two. When we reanalyze this study and only look at the women who were younger (within ten years of menopause) we find different results.

There was no increase in blood clots and there were benefits to the cardiovascular system.

In retrospect, what we have learned is that hormone replacement cannot remove health decline that has already taken place, but it can help to reduce the health decline after menopause.

4. The estrogen-only arm of the study showed benefits. In one part of the study, women were given a pill with estrogen (CEE) but without MPA. The women in this part of the study were found to have a decreased risk for heart disease and *no increased risk for breast cancer*. In fact, there was a trend toward a possible *decreased* risk for breast cancer. So why was this not all over the news?

Unfortunately, the increased risks with the combination pill became widely known, and hormone replacement therapy (HRT) was all lumped together with no differentiation between what *kind* of HRT women received.

Avoiding HRT based on this study is a disservice to women who are suffering with hormone deficiency symptoms, and it increases the risk and severity of age-related disease.

Let's learn more about estrogen.

There are actually several different kinds of estrogen:

Estrone (E1) is the estrogen that your body produces the most after menopause. High levels of estrone may actually lead to an **increased risk of breast cancer**.

Estradiol (E2) is the most potent form of estrogen. This is the main estrogen made by the ovaries during the premenopausal years. It is responsible for the growth of breasts and reproductive tissue. It also helps maintain bone density, maintains your memory, decreases fatigue, and prevents wrinkles by keeping skin hydrated. So when estradiol gets depleted, your body gets out of sync.

Estriol (E3) is thought to possibly **protect against breast cancer**. In Europe it is sometimes used to treat breast cancer. However, estriol does not seem to help protect your brain or heart as much as estradiol does. There are conflicting reports on whether estriol helps protect bones.

The goal of estrogen replacement is to prevent the symptoms and diseases associated with estrogen deficiency and optimize physical and mental function while minimizing risk.

Using the natural form of estrogen, avoiding oral estrogen, and carefully monitoring side effects of hormone excess appear to be the safest options available today.

It sounds like a lot to ask, but it is possible with bioidentical hormones under the guidance of an experienced physician.

Never heard of them? A brief explanation follows.

Bioidentical Hormones

Your ovaries make hormones. Bioidentical hormones are identical in molecular structure to those found in the human body. So, at least in theory, your body should not be able to tell whether the hormones came from your ovaries or the pharmacy.

Bioidentical estrogen is synthesized from plant compounds found in soy and wild yam. It is not possible to eat the soy or yam, or rub them on your skin, and get the same benefits.

In many parts of the world, bioidentical hormone replacement therapy (BHRT) is very common and widely accepted as standard practice. Experienced doctors feel comfortable with the safety profile of BHRT and large studies in Europe support that impression. Over the last thirty years, informed physicians have offered it to thousands of their patients.

In recent years, pharmaceutical companies have heard the message, and now more and more bioidentical estrogen preparations are FDA approved, available from regular pharmacies, and covered by health insurance.

Let's talk about some scientific concepts to explain why individually tailored dosing is preferable over one-size-fits-all dosing.

Our body's ability to process, use, and metabolize each hormone is unique to each person and is influenced by age, race, diet, genetics, environment, and other concurrent prescription drug use.

Imagine if the effective dose for you was very low compared to the average woman. You may experience symptoms of estrogen excess and suffer the results of the harmful byproducts we talked about earlier if you are prescribed a standard dose.

In fact, in the past when the one-size-fits-all approach to dosing was the only option, approximately 50 percent of women discontinued hormone replacement due to intolerable side effects.

There are many options for bioidentical estrogen, including individually customized creams (compounded BHRT); off-the-shelf FDA-approved patches, topical gel or spray; subcutaneous (under the skin) pellets; sublingual (under the tongue) lozenges; and pills. Each one should be considered with your doctor and the best option chosen, based on your symptoms and your lifestyle.

Here is a basic list of your options:

- **Estrogen patches.** A tiny patch is applied to the lower abdomen or buttocks once or twice weekly, allowing stable estrogen levels. Several doses are available.

  The disadvantage is that estrogen is the only bioidentical hormone available in a patch (there are some patches with bioidentical estrogen and a synthetic progestin).

  Some women develop a sensitivity to the adhesive over time, which causes itching and redness and the patches must be discontinued.

- **Estrogen pellets.** A tiny hormone pellet is implanted just below your skin during a quick, painless office procedure every three to four months. The pellets are smaller than a grain of rice and various doses are available.

The pellets dissolve completely, releasing a steady stream of hormone into your bloodstream. Of the various estrogen options, pellets allow the most stable hormone levels.

This is a very popular option because you don't have to remember to take something daily, and the results are very consistent.

- **Topical or vaginal cream.** Compounded or pharmaceutical creams and gels are rubbed on in the skin of the arms or legs or inserted vaginally once or twice daily.

  Compounded bioidentical estrogen is usually prescribed as *biest cream*, which is a combination of estriol and estradiol. Pharmaceutical versions have estradiol only.

  Some women like to apply the estrogen cream to their face to help prevent wrinkles and keep the glow in their skin.

- **Sublingual troches.** Troches are small, waxy lozenges that are dissolved under the tongue once or twice daily. The hormone is absorbed quickly into the bloodstream, and most of the liver metabolism is avoided. These are prepared by a compounding pharmacist and different flavors can be added.

  Compounded preparations have been somewhat controversial, as they are not FDA approved. It is not possible for them to be FDA approved, because each prescription is different, based on a woman's individual needs.

Compounded hormones are not better (after all, they are called *bioidentical* – so it should not matter whether the bioidentical estrogen comes from the pharmaceutical company or the compounding pharmacy).

The benefit of compounded hormones is that more doses are available, and it is possible to combine multiple hormones into one cream, allowing for more convenience of dosing and less expense.

• **Estrogen pills.** This choice is not considered optimal, as research shows that swallowing estrogen results in an increased risk of blood clots due to the effect on the liver. This risk can be avoided by choosing one of the other estrogen forms above.

All right, here's a question: if bioidentical estrogen replacement therapy is exactly what you are missing hormonally in your body, and it's easy to take, why isn't everyone doing it?

Pharmaceutical companies initially felt threatened by the idea of women using compounded hormones, and they helped to promote the idea that bioidentical hormones were not necessary.

In recent years, as research has shown the benefits of choosing bioidentical hormones, many bioidentical versions of estrogen have been developed by pharmaceutical companies that are available at your regular pharmacy, covered by your insurance.

One problem is that many healthcare providers are not aware that the hormones they are prescribing regularly ARE bioidentical (they don't know which are which).

Another problem is that often the term bioidentical is used to mean compounded hormones. Many doctors feel more comfortable with prescribing something that is made by a pharmaceutical company and are not familiar with using compounding pharmacies.

The fear of causing harm has been a major disincentive to prescribing hormones of any kind in the last decade. More and more research has been published since the WHI study that has shown the positive benefits of hormones, and we now understand more about the risks and how to minimize them.

The safest option available today seems to be taking the natural form of the hormones in the proper ratios, at physiologic doses, and in a proper delivery form.

In my opinion, bioidentical hormone therapy most closely replicates the physiologic estrogen production of our ovaries.

Remember, the goal with estrogen replacement is to help prevent the symptoms and diseases associated with estrogen deficiency and optimize physical and mental function while minimizing risk.

Making a decision about estrogen replacement is difficult when you receive conflicting messages. It is important that you understand all the factors before you proceed.

If you are considering BHRT, speak with a doctor experienced in all forms of hormone replacement, including bioidentical hormone therapy. Bioidentical hormone replacement may help you to get back to feeling normal again and may also help reduce the severity of age-related disease.

Chapter Six

I've Lost That Lovin' Feeling—
Testosterone Deficiency

Sue met her sister, Jill, at Starbucks on Saturday morning to catch up and discuss family plans for the upcoming holidays. Jill glanced across the table at her older sister and then leaned in a little closer, searching her eyes.

"Are you okay?" she asked. "You look tired."

Sue smiled half-heartedly. "Meet my new best friends, saggy and flabby," she joked, patting her sagging cheeks and belly respectively. "I think it finally happened. I'm old."

"Fifty is *not* old!" Jill rolled her eyes defiantly. "You still have lots of passion for life!"

Speaking of passion, Sue is embarrassed to admit that her formerly passionate relationship with her husband has come to a screaming halt—due to her total lack of interest in sex. He is confused, but trying to understand. Sue can only shrug her shoulders, because there seems to be no reason for her recent lack of interest.

* * *

Sue may be experiencing more than just aging; she may be suffering from low levels of testosterone. If elements of her story are true in your life, you too may have testosterone deficiency.

Testosterone deficiency is a real downer. Symptoms seem to center around a general lack of energy, saggy body, and blah emotions. You lack confidence and assertiveness. You feel like you're in a rut, and you don't snap out of it in a day or so.

A recent survey by the North American Menopause Society revealed that only 5 percent of women knew that women also produce testosterone naturally. Testosterone is responsible—more than estrogen—for women's sexual interest as well as vaginal lubrication upon arousal. Despite your best efforts, without adequate testosterone, there will be no fireworks.

Testosterone is produced in women by the ovaries and adrenal glands.

Quiz time!

Please answer YES or NO to the following questions:

Has your libido decreased?	YES	NO
Do you lack initiative?	YES	NO
Has your self-confidence lowered?	YES	NO
Have you lost your competitive drive?	YES	NO
Are you often tired?	YES	NO
Have you gained weight around your waist?	YES	NO
Have you lost muscle tone?	YES	NO
Do you have a hard time making decisions?	YES	NO

Are you depressed?	YES	NO
Are you less goal-oriented?	YES	NO
Is your skin more saggy?	YES	NO
Do you have vaginal dryness?	YES	NO
Is intercourse uncomfortable?	YES	NO
Are you having incontinence?	YES	NO

Add up the total number of times you answered YES to the questions above.

Total YES answers: _____

If you answered YES to fewer than five questions above, low testosterone may not be an issue for you.

If you answered YES to between five and seven questions above, you may be affected by low testosterone levels.

If you answered YES to eight or more of the questions above, it is likely that you suffer from testosterone deficiency.

Here is a more complete list of symptoms of testosterone deficiency:

- Thin lips
- Weight gain
- Anxiety
- Saggy cheeks
- Droopy eyelids
- Dry skin
- Low self-esteem
- Thinning hair

- Fatigue
- Loss of muscle tone
- Decreased libido
- Reduced competitive drive
- Weepiness or tendency to cry easily
- Lack of vaginal lubrication
- Lack of self confidence
- Urinary incontinence
- Lack of motivation

Estrogen and testosterone replacement work hand in hand. Remember, we women are a complex tapestry.

Is it just menopause that causes lower testosterone levels?

Actually, no.

Testosterone deficiency can occur at any age, due to many causes. Here are a few:

- **Birth control pills.** You may be taking a birth control pill that adversely affects the level of testosterone in your system. The synthetic estrogen in the pill reduces the amount of active testosterone available to your cells. Talk with your healthcare provider about options that may help to better balance your hormonal composition.

- **Depression.** Serious clinical depression—and here I mean not just the occasional blues—may cause testosterone deficiency. Testosterone levels rise and fall due to emotional as well as physical changes in the body. If you treat your depression, you may see testosterone levels begin to rise. Conversely, testosterone has antidepressant effects in women.

- **Psychological trauma.** Sometimes psychological trauma—such as the loss of a loved one or a serious car accident—may cause your testosterone levels to decrease. Working with a professional to resolve feelings associated with this trauma may bring your testosterone levels back to normal.

- **Childbirth.** If you recently gave birth, your body may now be producing less testosterone. Your doctor may suggest waiting a few months to see if these symptoms are temporary, and if testosterone levels will rise again on their own.

- **Chemotherapy.** If you have recently undergone chemotherapy treatments, your levels of testosterone may have decreased. Your doctor may prescribe a hormone treatment to help you regain the balance that was lost during your chemotherapy treatments.

- **Stress.** Sometimes too much stress can lead to burnout and lower testosterone levels. You may have to make some lifestyle changes in order to feel like yourself again or find other ways to alleviate your stress, such as exercise or getting more sleep.

- **HMG-CoA reductase inhibitors.** This is just a high-tech way to describe a group of prescription drugs, *statins*, that are used to lower cholesterol. While these drugs will lower cholesterol, they may also lower testosterone levels.

- **Endometriosis.** If you suffer from this disease, you may also have lower testosterone levels. If this is the case, some of the treatments listed below may help you restore the hormones that have been lost.

- **Hysterectomy.** More than 30 percent of adult women in America have undergone removal of their uterus. Leaving your ovaries intact does not guarantee they will work normally. It is not uncommon to have earlier menopausal symptoms after a hysterectomy, including testosterone deficiency.

- **Oophorectomy (removal of the ovaries).** Fifty percent of your testosterone is made in your ovaries. If you have your ovaries removed for any reason, you have a high chance of become testosterone deficient.

- **Hormone replacement therapy.** If you are taking estrogen pills, they can reduce the amount of active testosterone available. You may want to consider another form of estrogen replacement, such as transdermal patches, creams, or pellet therapy.

By the time most women reach age forty, they are producing half as much testosterone as they were in their twenties.

For both women and men, the drop in testosterone varies from person to person. Some women may not experience any real symptoms when testosterone levels decrease. Other women feel like they have turned into some sort of alien when testosterone levels plummet. They feel emotionally and physically out of whack.

Another interesting point to note is that women who normally have fairly high levels of testosterone in their system and experience a radical drop, possibly as a result of chemotherapy or a hysterectomy, may be much more uncomfortable with the change than women who go through their entire life with generally lower levels of testosterone.

If you are experiencing many of the symptoms listed above, you can get help. Talk with your doctor about how you can restore some of the testosterone that is no longer being produced in your body.

Adding testosterone is not unfeminine or unseemly. It may help you return your body to a more comfortable hormonal level. It may even help you recapture some of the energy and libido of your youth.

Studies show that women with surgical menopause who were treated with both estrogen and testosterone together experienced improvements in both sexual energy and sense of well-being compared to those not treated with anything and those treated with estrogen alone.

It is unfortunately common that hormones are not addressed and women are placed on antidepressants first.

Many treatments for menopause concentrate on increasing estrogen levels. However, we have already established that no one hormone works alone. Your hormones are a complex and intricate system. Physicians have found that adding testosterone, even in very small doses, helps to increase the positive effects of estrogen, progesterone, and other hormones in your body.

Testosterone promotes metabolic efficiency. It can exert influence on nearly every cell in the body.

Testosterone has also been shown to improve your sex drive, increase energy, and increase bone strength—something that does not necessarily happen by adding estrogen alone.

Studies confirm that combining testosterone and estrogen in women not only prevents bone loss, but significantly increases bone density.

Also, testosterone acts with estrogen to help preserve memory. So, small amounts of testosterone should be considered in the hormone cocktail that you and your doctor come up with to combat the symptoms of menopause.

How do you know for sure if you have a testosterone deficiency?

There are several ways you can find out for certain if your testosterone levels are low.

Your healthcare provider can perform a test to measure your testosterone levels in blood, saliva, or urine to help you get to the real cause of your symptoms.

Remember to look at social issues as well as physical issues when discussing testosterone levels. The levels of testosterone in your body go up and down throughout the day for a number of reasons.

Here are a few additional observations:

- Testosterone levels are highest in the morning, and by the end of the day, they can fall to half of what they were.

- Testosterone levels rise and fall with successes and failures that you experience throughout the day.

- Sexual experiences create a rise in testosterone. This happens more for women than men.

Say you take the test, and it confirms that your testosterone levels are low. You are suffering from several of the symptoms mentioned above, and you really want to get back to normal.

What can you do to get testosterone levels to go back up, short of turning back the clock?

If you are suffering from testosterone deficiency, you have a number of options for restoring testosterone levels.

Avoid oral testosterone and synthetic testosterone. Studies have shown that these may cause liver toxicity or even liver tumors.

Options for testosterone replacement include:

- **Transdermal cream or gel** from the compounding pharmacist may be applied to the skin of the arms or legs once or twice daily. It also may be applied vaginally or externally to the clitoral area.

- **Testosterone troches** (lozenges that dissolve under the tongue) are used once or twice daily. These are absorbed directly into the bloodstream.

- **Testosterone pellets** are a very popular option. A tiny pellet (approximately the size of a grain of rice) is inserted under the skin of the upper buttock during a quick, painless office procedure. The pellets slowly dissolve over the next three months and provide a very stable release of testosterone directly into the bloodstream.

  Testosterone pellet therapy has been used since the 1930s and research has shown benefits to bone health, reduction in migraine headaches, improved PMS symptoms, as well as improved energy, mood, and libido.

It typically takes a very small amount of testosterone to have a very large effect in women, because testosterone levels in women are much lower than in men.

Now, let's throw another layer onto the puzzle:
Dehydroepiandrosterone.

It sounds very complicated, and the name comes close to using every letter in the alphabet. So, let's go with DHEA from here on out.

DHEA is a hormone made in the adrenal glands. The adrenal glands sit on top of the kidneys and are responsible for making your major stress hormones, including adrenaline; hence the name.

DHEA is used to make testosterone and estrogen in women and men. DHEA declines over your lifetime. By age seventy, you will probably be making only one-fourth of the DHEA you made in your teens.

Now you're getting the connection, aren't you?

DHEA has several functions, many of which are similar to testosterone:

- Increases bone health
- Promotes weight loss
- Increases brain function
- Decreases cholesterol
- Decreases fatty deposits
- Supports the immune system
- Helps you deal with stress
- Increases sense of well-being
- Decreases allergic reactions

Since DHEA is a precursor to testosterone, increasing DHEA is another way of elevating your testosterone. The replacement of DHEA produces parallel results.

It improves your quality of life by reversing the effects of stress, improving sleep, increasing your brain function and immune system function, increasing your sense of well-being, decreasing joint stiffness, and increasing muscle strength.

DHEA may be a slightly more gentle way of increasing your testosterone levels, and it is available in pill or cream form without a prescription in the United States.

DHEA pills are commonly available in doses of twenty-five to fifty milligrams. The typical starting dose for women is only five milligrams. You read that right. Most pills are too strong and will likely result in side effects like oily skin and acne. There are now a few companies making pills in the smaller formulation, but you may need to shop around.

Speak with your doctor about the relationship between DHEA and testosterone if you find that your testosterone levels are low. Keep in mind that women need a much lower dosage of DHEA than men. A little bit goes a long way in the female body.

Even supplements thought of as natural hormones can be dangerous if taken in the wrong dosage or combined with prescription medications. And there is no benefit to taking DHEA if your levels are NOT low to begin with.

Consult with your doctor if you decide to take any natural supplements, so you don't end up feeling worse, rather than better. Make sure that once DHEA is started, your levels are followed.

The moral of the story is:

You may have testosterone deficiency if you suffer from the symptoms mentioned in this chapter. If test results prove that you do, take steps to realign your hormonal balance.

You can do this in a number of ways, including replacing what you have lost through hormone replacement. You—and your significant other—may be thrilled with the results!

Chapter Seven

Am I Going to Grow Hair on My Chest?
Testosterone Excess

Forty-eight-year-old Jane glared at the half-eaten chocolate doughnut making a greasy hole in the napkin on the corner of her desk.

Here we go again, she thought. Is this going to be another day of bouncing back and forth between sugar cravings and a taste for salt? I wonder if I could bribe the janitor into removing all vending machines from this floor?

Jane usually stuck to a relatively healthy diet, but lately her cravings were getting the best of her. That wasn't all. Five minutes earlier she had let her anger get the best of her, too, as she chewed out a subordinate before dismissing him from her office.

Where did that anger come from?

Jane felt as though she had lost all patience, and the smallest infraction caused her irritation to boil over into borderline rage.

Earlier that morning, Jane noticed what looked like peach fuzz growing on her upper lip as she was applying her makeup. She grimaced into the mirror.

Is this what happens when I play with the big boys? she thought. Am I turning into a caveman? What's next, hair on my chest?

Jane's anger and unwanted hair growth is most likely not a side effect of a promotion in a male-dominated office. However, chances are she is suffering from testosterone excess.

Remember, testosterone has a lot of positive benefits, such as:

- Maintains bone strength
- Increases interest in sex
- Maintains memory
- Decreases body fat
- Increases muscle strength
- Increases a sense of well-being
- Increases motivation and competitive drive
- Helps to maintain skin elasticity, as opposed to saggy skin

Well, that all sounds great. You would probably enjoy an increased sex drive and non-saggy skin, right? Testosterone is important to women as well as men, but only at much lower levels. So if you are suffering from excess testosterone, it's not so great.

Let's take the quiz.

Please answer YES or NO to the following questions:

Have you experienced balding or thinning hair?   YES   NO

Do you have acne?   YES   NO

Have your periods stopped or become irregular?   YES   NO

Is hair growing on your face, neck, chest,
    or abdomen?   YES   NO

Do you anger easily?	YES	NO
Have you experienced salt or sugar cravings?	YES	NO
Do you perspire more easily?	YES	NO
Do you have more body odor recently?	YES	NO
Do you have oily skin?	YES	NO
Do you have oily hair?	YES	NO

Add up the number of times you answered YES to the questions above.

Total YES answers: _____

If you answered YES to fewer than four of the questions above, excess testosterone is not likely to be an issue for you.

If you answered YES to between four and six of the questions above, you may be experiencing excess testosterone levels.

If you answered YES to seven or more of the questions above, it is likely that you are experiencing testosterone excess.

Testosterone plays at least five major roles in the body for women and men:

1. It regulates mood.

2. It builds energy.

3. It increases libido.

4. It is critical for maintaining weight.

5. Excess levels cause development of masculine traits.

Women produce a small amount of testosterone in the ovaries and in the adrenal glands to aid in developing the first four of the above traits. However, abnormally high levels of testosterone in women can produce a number of unwanted symptoms.

Here is a more comprehensive list of symptoms and signs of excess testosterone:

- Weight gain
- Acne
- Facial hair
- Chest hair
- Insulin resistance (prediabetes)
- Anxiety
- Increased risk of heart disease
- Fatigue
- Hypoglycemia (low blood sugar)
- Hair loss in the scalp
- Salt and sugar cravings
- Anger and agitation
- Depression
- Oily skin
- Ovarian cysts
- Infertility
- Irregular periods

What can you do to change the hormonal balance and lower your testosterone levels?

First, there are a few natural steps you can try to see if testosterone levels will go down. If you are a smoker, this would be a good time to try quitting. Also, limit your alcohol consumption or use of recreational drugs. Cigarettes, alcohol, and other recreational drugs can adversely affect your hormonal balance.

Saw palmetto is an herbal nutritional supplement that can be somewhat helpful. It helps to reduce the conversion of testosterone into its even more potent metabolite, dihydrotestosterone (DHT). DHT is three times more powerful than testosterone, so reducing this strong hormone may result in decreased symptoms.

Insulin resistance (prediabetes) is very common in women in the United States. There is a relationship between insulin and testosterone.

The higher levels of insulin found in prediabetic women trigger more testosterone production. Testosterone causes more insulin resistance. So a feed-forward cycle is created, resulting in the symptoms of too much insulin *and* too much testosterone. Treatments aimed at improving insulin function can also help lower testosterone.

Eating a healthy diet of whole, unprocessed foods and reducing the amount of processed carbohydrates (the white stuff: sugar, bread, pasta, rice, potatoes) can help. Avoiding the unhealthy trans fats found in deep-fried foods and commercially prepared baked goods like some cookies and crackers is also important, as this type of fat increases problems with insulin. See the chapter on insulin for more information.

Losing weight helps improve insulin function and may result in improved testosterone levels.

Medications are sometimes needed in more severe cases. Metformin is a medication used to improve insulin function. Spironolactone is a medication that blocks the effects of testosterone and is often used to reduce acne and excess hair growth.

The standard treatment in many medical offices is to prescribe birth control pills. Because these reduce the active levels of testosterone, they can reduce the symptoms of excess testosterone in women who need contraceptives.

Often, with a holistic approach, similar benefits can be seen without needing to prescribe birth control pills.

Women who have high testosterone levels often do not ovulate regularly, which results in low progesterone levels. Progesterone also helps to reduce the conversion of testosterone into the stronger DHT, and replacing natural progesterone can help reduce symptoms of testosterone excess in some women.

Unfortunately, as we are all unique, occasionally some women convert progesterone into more testosterone and symptoms such as acne may actually increase instead of improving. A physician skilled in the use of BHRT can help determine the best approach for you.

Chapter Eight

Stressed and Tired—
Adrenal Fatigue

Brenda sat on the couch half-heartedly dangling a large spoon in a half-eaten pint of ice cream. She was halfway through her second *Dallas* rerun on the Soap Channel.

Now, you would think bad hair and big shoulder pads would put me right to sleep, she thought, but nope. Here I am again. On the couch with my friends Ben & Jerry at 11 p.m.

Brenda had been experiencing increasing bouts of insomnia for the last several months, ever since the stress level in her job skyrocketed.

She was living on coffee by day and ice cream and chocolate by night, while working like a mad woman at least six days a week. She was tired of fearing for her job; tired of being pulled in twelve different directions at work; tired of the rat race. She was exhausted from the moment she woke up until about 6 p.m.

Had the stress finally gotten the best of her? Brenda felt like she was walking through molasses. It took at least a venti coffee to get her going in the morning. The world was moving at light speed, but she felt like she just couldn't keep up.

* * *

Brenda may be suffering from adrenal fatigue.

Chronic stress is very common—almost expected—in our modern world. Stress is a likely component in the lives of successful, driven, type A individuals. Adrenal fatigue occurs when stress overrides the body's ability to compensate and recover.

Adrenal fatigue is a disorder that can affect anyone who is under prolonged physical or emotional stress. It is now known that adrenal fatigue can contribute to other health issues, such as obesity, allergies, or asthma.

Adrenal fatigue very often goes undiagnosed, because its symptoms are part of everyday life for so many individuals in the twenty-first century.

Take a quiz to see if you share any of Brenda's symptoms of adrenal fatigue.

Please answer YES or NO to the following questions:

Do you have a hard time getting up
   in the morning?   YES   NO

Do you have a drop in energy
   in the late afternoon?   YES   NO

Do you have hair loss?   YES   NO

Do you have low blood pressure?   YES   NO

If you stand up quickly, do you feel like
   you might pass out?   YES   NO

Do you get recurrent infections?   YES   NO

Are you under a lot of emotional stress?	YES	NO
Have you lost your sex drive?	YES	NO
Are you sensitive to light and noise?	YES	NO
Do you have panic attacks?	YES	NO
Do you crave salt or sugar?	YES	NO
Do you feel like you need caffeine to make it through the day?	YES	NO
Do you no longer enjoy things you used to enjoy?	YES	NO
Do you have more difficulty coping with stressful situations?	YES	NO
Do you feel tired after exercising?	YES	NO

If you answered YES to fewer than five of the questions above, you probably are not suffering from adrenal fatigue.

If you answered YES to between five and seven of the questions above, you may be experiencing adrenal fatigue.

If you answered YES to eight or more of the questions above, it is likely that you are experiencing adrenal fatigue.

Your adrenal glands are located above the kidneys, and their main responsibility is to regulate the body's stress by synthesizing hormones, including cortisol and adrenaline. If something requires your fight-or-flight response to kick in, it's up to the adrenal glands to call out the troops and get the necessary hormones going to help you respond.

In a healthy person, the adrenal glands work with remarkable precision. If a stressful situation arises, the following things will happen almost simultaneously:

- You heart rate will increase.

- Your energy that has been stored will be immediately released for use.

- Digestion will slow down.

- Blood pressure will increase.

- All secondary functions will slow down, so you can give your full attention to the problem.

- Your senses will immediately become very acute.

However, it takes an incredible amount of energy to mobilize this army. Can you imagine what it would be like if your body was under this kind of stress for prolonged periods of time? It would be like constantly blowing the horn to rally the troops for battle.

Adrenal fatigue happens when the adrenal glands finally hit overload, and they are unable to continue to produce stress hormones efficiently.

It is estimated that more than 80 percent of the people in North America suffer from adrenal fatigue. Most often it goes undiagnosed.

Why?

Because stress is a normal part of our society, it is not considered a real medical problem. You may realize that you have stress, but you don't think about the real physical toll stress can take on your body.

Some people who suffer from the physical affects of stress will go from doctor to doctor and be told that they are just fine.

They end up feeling like a hypochondriac, because there are no tangible reasons for feeling a little under the weather or tired or just plain rundown.

Individuals suffering from adrenal fatigue seem to have great difficulty getting up in the morning, even if they went to bed at a reasonable hour. They are tired for no obvious reason and feel overwhelmed and rundown. They have trouble coping with stress.

Women with adrenal fatigue may also crave salty or sweet snacks, and they have difficulty bouncing back from a cold or illness. Often they finally feel awake and alert in the evening, and then have difficulty falling asleep.

Here are a few additional symptoms of adrenal fatigue:

- Hypoglycemia (drop in blood sugar)
- Digestive problems
- Decreased libido
- Low blood pressure
- Nervousness
- Low body temperature
- Allergies
- Decreased ability to handle stress
- Thin and dry skin
- Hair loss
- Pain in upper back or neck
- Feel better suddenly after a meal
- Memory loss
- Feel unrefreshed in the morning even after adequate sleep

What causes adrenal fatigue?

The number one factor is **chronic stress**. The function of the adrenal glands is to help in emergency situations. It is important to remember two very important items related to those situations:

1. When the adrenal glands go into fight-or-flight mode, everything else going on in your body is pretty much put on hold. Once the adrenal glands start producing cortisol to combat stress, all other metabolic functions slow down.

2. This kind of adrenal gland function isn't meant to go on for a prolonged period of time. It is a short-term, rapid-fire, instant response. It is meant to last about as long as a sprint, not a marathon.

So, when stress is constant in your life, the adrenal glands may over-function and burn out, causing adrenal fatigue. Moving, changing jobs, the death of a loved one, losing a job, marital problems, or chronic illness may contribute to a constant level of stress that could result in adrenal fatigue.

Here is a list of common stressors that may lead to adrenal fatigue:

- Excessive exercise (yes, you really can over-train)
- Depression
- Too much sugar
- Too much caffeine
- Anger
- Low blood sugar
- Yo-yo dieting
- Prolonged fear

- Financial instability
- Sleep deprivation
- Guilt
- Fear of losing a job
- Surgery
- Lowgrade infections
- Hidden food sensitivities

When your body tries to fight an infection, you experience fatigue. That is because most of your resources are taking on the infection to try to boot it out of the neighborhood.

Some infections can occur without any obvious outward signs at first. Gastrointestinal infections, like *Candida albicans* (a type of yeast) is an example.

Hidden food sensitivities are even more common—possibly up to one in three women has this problem. You can develop sensitivities to common healthy foods—when you eat the food, your immune system reacts, causing inflammation and fatigue.

Both infections and food sensitivities are what we consider to be stresses on your system, even if you are not aware of the problems.

Toxins in the environment, allergies, chronic pain, and health conditions such as fibromyalgia or hypothyroidism are all examples of physical stressors that can also affect your adrenal gland function and cortisol levels.

So, if you are exhibiting many of the symptoms of extreme fatigue listed above, but you don't think emotional stress is the reason, you may want to look into some of these factors as the cause.

Cortisol is produced by the adrenal glands, and it is one of the only hormones that *increases* rather than decreases as you get older. It also increases in the early stages of adrenal fatigue.

Three main things send cortisol production into high gear:

1. Stress
2. Depression
3. Chronic inflammation

Cortisol has many functions in the body:

- Balances your blood sugar
- Helps you to fall asleep at night and awaken in the morning
- Controls weight
- Balances your mood
- Regulates your immune system
- Regulates the other hormones, such as testosterone, estrogen, DHEA, and insulin

So, how is that bad?

Elevated cortisol can actually have a negative effect on your system. If your levels of cortisol remain high for a long period of time, cortisol can actually start to tear your body down, rather than build it up.

Here are a few consequences of high levels of cortisol:

- Irritability
- Weight gain
- Shakiness between meals
- Cravings for sugar
- Binge eating
- Increased blood pressure

- Low energy
- Easy bruising
- Increased infections
- Bone loss
- High blood sugar
- Poor memory
- Loss of muscle mass

Cortisol levels spike as the adrenal glands try to combat stress or infection, and if there is no relief, eventually your adrenal glands run out of gas. Exhaustion occurs, and levels of cortisol drop.

There is another way that chronically elevated cortisol levels can cause you to run out of steam. Excess cortisol is toxic to the brain — it literally causes brain shrinkage. As a self-defense mechanism, the brain can shut down cortisol production, like blowing a fuse or tripping a breaker on an electrical panel.

When your adrenal function is depressed, DHEA levels will be reduced as well. Remember: DHEA is a precursor to the production of estrogen, testosterone, and progesterone. So, if it drops, the balance of other hormones in the body quickly breaks down. A decrease in DHEA also means the following could happen:

- Bone density loss
- Fatigue
- Decreased interest in sex
- Achy joints
- Loss of muscle tone
- Depression
- Lower immune system function

If the adrenal glands remain out of sync and are not normalized, you will eventually end up with adrenal fatigue.

How do you know if you really have adrenal fatigue, and you're not just tired and grouchy?

Take a test to find out. Be sure to find a healthcare provider who is knowledgeable about adrenal fatigue. Most understand what to do if the adrenal gland is completely shot, but few assess the stages before complete failure.

The easiest way is to test saliva or urine at different times of the day to find out what your cortisol levels are.

The ideal adrenal health results show higher levels of cortisol in the morning (to give you energy to hop out of bed and get started with your day); lower but steady levels throughout the rest of the day; and declining levels at night, so that you can easily relax and go to sleep.

If your cortisol levels are signaling the early stages of adrenal fatigue, you may maintain high levels throughout the day, and they may even go up in the evening.

Finally, if you are definitely suffering from adrenal fatigue, your levels of cortisol will remain at the low end of normal level all day. That is because your adrenal glands were overworked for so long that they finally gave up.

Are you wondering whether or not you should go to the trouble of getting a panel of tests?

You probably do **not** need to test your hormonal levels if:

- You feel generally happy.

- Your emotions do not shift dramatically throughout the day.

- You get between seven and nine hours of sleep most nights.

- You wake up feeling well-rested.

- You are able to maintain a healthy weight.

- Your energy level seems to stay pretty steady throughout the day.

On the other hand, you may want to consider testing your hormonal levels with a panel of tests if:

- You feel like your emotions are all over the map.

- You depend on some sort of caffeine to get going and maintain your energy level throughout the day. ✓

- You generally don't sleep well and can't remember when you got a full seven hours of sleep.

- You can't seem to lose weight, even after trying numerous fad diets. ✓

- You have carbohydrate or sugar cravings, especially when you are in emotional distress.

- You have to drag yourself out of bed in the morning. ✓

So, if you and your doctor come to the conclusion that you are suffering from adrenal fatigue, how can you reverse the cycle and get your adrenal glands to normalize?

Here are seven steps you can take right now:

1. **Remove or manage stress.** Deal with the issues that are causing you stress in order to alleviate the problems. Consider yoga, breathing exercises, visualization, meditation, and prayer.

2. **Sleep.** Try to get to sleep by ten o'clock every night. Why is that the magic hour? If you stay up past 11 p.m., your adrenal glands kick in to help you stay awake. This puts stress on your system and starts a cycle you do not want to continue.

   Strive for at least eight hours of sleep each night. If you keep your bedtime consistent, your body will eventually get used to the routine and you will feel sleepy around 10 p.m.

3. **Avoid caffeine.** Try herbal tea instead of caffeinated beverages. Caffeine is a stimulant, and it results in similar effects as stress. So it makes you feel better for a few hours, but in the long run it is making things worse.

4. **Turn off the TV.** The light from TVs and especially computer monitors tricks your brain into thinking it is still daytime. Experiment with turning off the TV and your computer by eight o'clock each night and see if it is easier to fall asleep.

5. **Exercise.** You don't have to go crazy and get a personal trainer with a death wish. Just twenty to thirty minutes a day is great.

   Try to balance aerobic exercise, strength training (weights), and flexibility. Exercise reduces stress, increases blood flow, and also helps to normalize your hormone levels.

   If you are having trouble falling asleep, exercising earlier in the day is probably the best bet.

If you are really exhausted, gentle exercise like yoga or tai chi is best. You should feel better after exercise, not so tired that you want to go home for a nap.

6. **Talk to your healthcare provider about nutritional supplements.** There are a number of herbs that can help support adrenal function. These are known as herbal *adaptogens*, and have been used for thousands of years all over the world to help cope with stress. Some examples are Rhodiola, ashwagandha, and cordyceps (a genus of mushroom).

7. **Adjust your eating patterns.** Do not skip breakfast, even if you're not hungry. Grab some peanut butter and an apple, anything to get your system going in the morning.

    Five small meals throughout the day to help stabilize blood sugar levels seem to have a better overall effect on the body than the traditional three large meals.

Tell your healthcare providers about any supplements you are taking, in case there is a possibility that they may counteract other treatments.

Remember that with adrenal fatigue, your entire hormone balance can be disrupted. Using the above measures can help and you may feel better quickly, but it may take six months or longer before the full benefits are appreciated.

If you are suffering from adrenal fatigue, take some time to take care of yourself:

- Get more sleep.

- Make sure your diet is healthy.

- Exercise.

- Laugh.

- Do something every day that makes you happy.

- Try to resolve issues that are causing major stress in your life.

Simple changes in your daily life may make all the difference to your health and well-being.

If symptoms persist, speak with your healthcare practitioner about further tests to see if infection or other issues may be at the root of your problem.

Chapter Nine

Moving in Slo-Mo—
Thyroid Deficiency

Nancy leaned against the counter in her sister Ruth's kitchen while the enticing smells of Thanksgiving turkey hung heavy in the room. Ruth was basting the bird one last time.

"I do not know what is up with me lately," Nancy complained, lazily picking up her glass of chardonnay and taking a sip. "I feel like one of those balloons in the Macy's Thanksgiving Day Parade."

Ruth laughed and shut the oven door.

"I'm serious! This is so embarrassing, but if I can't tell you, who can I tell?" Nancy leaned toward her sister conspiratorially. "I am soooo bloated, I can hardly breathe. I've gained weight; I'm retaining water; I'm constipated all the time; my face is puffy; and I have the get-up-and-go of a turtle. I feel like I'm living my life in slo-mo."

"Maybe it's just a little irregularity." Ruth patted Nancy's hand.

"But it's not going away! I feel like Tom Turkey in there. Any minute now, my little button is gonna pop out and announce, 'She's done! Stick a fork in her! This old bird can't possibly expand any more.' "

* * *

Nancy probably has not turned into a human Macy's parade balloon. She may be suffering from thyroid deficiency.

Let's go right to the quiz this time. This is a lengthy one.

Please answer YES or NO to the following questions:

Is your voice hoarse?	(YES)	NO
Is your blood pressure low?	(YES)	NO
Do you have difficulty forming thoughts?	(YES)	NO
Are you often tired?	(YES)	NO
Do you have difficulty sleeping?	(YES)	NO
Do you have joint pain?	(YES)	NO
Is your skin pasty and pale?	(YES)	NO
Do you have a slow pulse rate?	(YES)	NO
Do you have periods of depression?	YES	(NO)
Do you have high cholesterol?	(YES)	NO
Do you have cold hands and feet?	(YES)	NO
Do your muscles ache?	(YES)	NO
Do you have sleep apnea?	? YES	NO
Is it hard for you to lose weight?	(YES)	NO
Have you experienced scalp hair loss?	? YES	NO
Do you have dry skin?	(YES)	NO
Does your skin get itchy in the winter?	(YES)	NO

Do you have recurrent headaches? YES ~~NO~~

Is your tongue enlarged? (YES) NO

Does your body temperature run below 98.6°F? (YES) NO

Has your body hair decreased? (YES) NO

Is your face puffy? YES (NO)

Are your eyelids swollen? (YES) NO

Do you have less than one bowel
movement per day? (YES) NO

Are you sensitive to the cold? (YES) NO

Do you have poor short-term memory? (YES) NO

Are you still tired when you get up
in the morning? (YES) NO

Have you had problems with infertility
or miscarriages? YES (NO)

Do you get tired in the afternoon? (YES) NO

Are you retaining fluid? (YES) NO

Do you have tingling in your hands and feet? (YES) NO

Are your eyebrows and eyelashes thinning? (YES) NO

Do you sweat less than you used to? (YES) NO

Are you easily susceptible to infection? (YES) NO

If you answered YES to fewer than six of the questions above, there may be another reason besides low thyroid function for your symptoms.

If you answered YES to between six and fifteen questions above, you may be experiencing thyroid deficiency.

If you answered YES to more than fifteen questions above, there is a good chance you have low thyroid function.

Obviously from the number of questions asked this time, there are a quite a few symptoms associated with thyroid deficiency, or hypothyroidism. Women are much more likely to have hypothyroidism than men.

The thyroid gland is shaped like a butterfly, and it is located in your throat. Its main function is to produce hormones that regulate metabolism.

The thyroid takes iodine (which is obtained mostly from foods like seafood and iodized salt) and converts it to hormones. The most important hormone it produces is T4 (thyroxine). The other important thyroid hormone, T3 (triiodothyronine), is made in your tissues, where T4 gets converted into T3.

Thyroid hormones set your metabolic rate (the rate at which you burn calories). They also set your internal thermostat (your body temperature).

Thyroid levels are affected by the levels of other hormones, especially progesterone and cortisol.

As we have already learned, thyroid hormones have a huge impact on your overall health. They impact all aspects of your metabolism, as well as your heart rate, muscle growth, bone health, and cholesterol level.

Lack of thyroid hormones can cause depression, weight gain, sluggishness, and even heart failure.

If your body is not producing enough thyroid hormone, the delicate chemical balance tips, and your tapestry starts to unravel. Symptoms of thyroid deficiency are not seen right away, but eventually health problems start to pop up if hypothyroidism is not treated.

The following is a more complete list of symptoms of thyroid deficiency or hypothyroidism:

- Weight gain/hard to lose weight
- Moving slowly
- Slow heart rate
- Slow speech
- Stiffness in the morning
- Muscle pain
- Joint pain
- Muscle cramps
- Muscle weakness
- Constipation
- Fluid retention
- Swollen legs, feet, abdomen, hands
- Irregular menstruation
- Poor circulation
- Low body temperature
- Low blood pressure
- Cold hands and feet
- Intolerance of cold
- Yellowish skin
- Dry skin
- Dry bumps on the skin of the upper arms and thighs
- Brittle nails
- Coarse, dry hair
- Hair loss

- Husky or hoarse voice ✓
- Droopy eyelids
- Swollen eyelids
- Fatigue ✓
- Depression
- Easily agitated ✓
- Lack of interest in sex
- Inability to concentrate ✓
- Panic attacks
- Insomnia

One of the side effects of low thyroid hormones is high cholesterol. In the United States, high cholesterol is often treated with medication; however, the real problem may not be addressed. Thyroid deficiency may be the underlying cause.

The most common cause of hypothyroidism in the United States is Hashimoto's thyroiditis. It is characterized by an immune system that gets mixed up and starts making antibodies that attack the thyroid gland, causing damage.

What else can go wrong with thyroid function?

Lets talk about the complicated interplay of the different types of thyroid hormones.

T4 is made in the thyroid gland. It circulates in your bloodstream, but it doesn't actually do much. When it gets to the level of your tissues, you have to convert it into T3, which is where all the action is. T3 attaches to your cells and tells them to burn more calories, generate more energy, heat you up, and get things moving.

If you are deficient in certain important nutrients, like zinc and selenium, then you may not convert T4 into T3 properly.

Chronic stress is another cause of poor T4 to T3 conversion.

In these cases, your thyroid gland is doing its job just fine — but your cells aren't getting enough of the activating signal (T3), so you don't *feel* fine.

So, you can see that there are a number of reasons why you could feel like you are hypothyroid, yet be told that your thyroid level is normal.

How do we test for hypothyroidism?

The most common screening blood test measures TSH (Thyroid Stimulating Hormone) levels. If your TSH is high, it means you are hypothyroid (your thyroid gland is not functioning well enough). Full-blown hypothyroidism will be picked up by this test.

Remember, the TSH levels will be HIGH if your thyroid function is *low* — this can get very confusing!

You may have symptoms of low thyroid, but be told by your doctor that your thyroid is normal because you have a normal TSH level.

The normal range for TSH is a little controversial right now. There is a very wide range of what constitutes normal, and different labs set different limits. It is possible to test normal with one lab and outside of the normal range at another lab.

If you have symptoms of hypothyroidism but your TSH levels register as normal, make sure that you also include a free T3 and free T4 test in the blood test. If free T3 or free T4 is low, there is a problem.

A newer test is Reverse T3. This is a blocking thyroid hormone, so you don't want too much of this one. It can go up if you have chronic inflammation, chronic stress, or digestive problems, making you feel like you don't have enough thyroid function.

There are also tests to measure for antibodies that are attacking your thyroid gland (TPO antibodies). This is how we can tell whether the cause of your problem is Hashimoto's or not.

If you are being treated with synthetic T4 therapy and still have symptoms, make sure that all of the labs are tested. It is quite possible that you are not converting the T4 in your pill into the T3 that your cells need, and maybe it is being converted into too much Reverse T3 instead.

This is a very common scenario. Your TSH is normal, and your doctor is very happy with your dose, even though you still have all the symptoms of low thyroid. If this is the problem for you, a change in treatment can make all the difference.

Let's talk treatments.

Treatment usually starts with synthetic T4 hormones, such as Synthroid and Levoxyl. Typically, low doses are initially started and the dose is raised until the symptoms resolve and lab test results normalize.

In some cases, symptoms persist even after treatment with synthetic T4 hormones.

There are several reasons why thyroid function may be diminished in the face of normal tests:

- The test results may be "normal" but not "optimal."

- There may be a problem converting the inactive form of thyroid (T4) to the active form (T3).

- There may be a problem with how T3 attaches to cells and delivers its message to increase metabolism.

Thyroid levels are affected by the levels of other hormones, especially estrogen, progesterone, and cortisol, so addressing the other hormone levels is important.

Are there any natural treatments for hypothyroidism?

Yes, there are.

Dessicated thyroid is a prescription medication derived from freeze-dried porcine (pig) thyroid tissue. It contains both T4 and T3 (as well as other natural factors).

It is available as a generic as well as several different brand names (Armour, Naturethroid, WPthyroid). It has been approved for use in the United States since 1939, but had fallen out of favor when newer, synthetic thyroid preparations came on the market.

Dessicated thyroid is preferred by most of my patients because it often alleviates more symptoms than synthetic T4.

Since every one of us is different, the best approach may be to try one route and continue to monitor changes in your body with symptoms and blood tests. Then, you and your doctor may adjust your therapy as needed.

Are there any nutrients that will enhance thyroid function?

Yes. Here is a list of some of the nutrients that may help increase your thyroid function:

- **Iodine.** Iodine is essential for producing thyroid hormone. Low iodine levels can produce goiter (an abnormal swelling of the thyroid gland) or hypothyroidism.

There seems to be a relationship between hypothyroidism and breast cancer, and iodine may have an integral part in that relationship. Women in Japan have high levels of iodine, probably due to their environment and diet. They also have a very low rate of breast cancer.

Once an iodine deficiency is corrected, some patients with hypothyroidism find they can lower their dose of thyroid hormone.

There is a lot of controversy over how prevalent iodine deficiency is in the United States. Iodine tests are now available to help determine whether or not this is a good option for you to try.

It is important to use caution with iodine in women with Hashimoto's, as iodine can cause them to develop hyperthyroidism.

- **Iron.** Iron is essential for normal thyroid hormone metabolism. A simple blood test done by your doctor can determine if you are deficient in iron. If this is the case, increasing your iron intake may help increase your overall thyroid hormone level.

- **Zinc.** The latest research points to the fact that zinc may play an important role in thyroid hormone function and thus in your overall metabolism. Zinc may make a significant contribution to the conversion of T4 to T3 hormones. So, if your zinc levels are low, try supplementing them to see if some of your hypothyroidism symptoms decrease.

- **Selenium.** Selenium is a required ingredient for thyroid activation, synthesis, and metabolism. If levels of selenium are low, the conversion of T4 to T3 could be reduced.

Studies have also shown that thyroiditis symptoms were significantly reduced after selenium supplements were added to patients' diets and that levels of anti-thyroid antibodies may be reduced.

If you are suffering from hypothyroidism, speak with your doctor about being tested for your nutrient status, and whether taking some of these supplements may be appropriate for you. Then monitor your symptoms and follow up with additional blood tests to find out if your thyroid hormone levels improve.

Remember that it is important for you to work with your healthcare provider to make sure that you are taking the right supplements in the right dosages.

Chapter Ten

Should I be Worried?
Insulin Resistance

Judy was fifty-four years old and was beginning to feel a little worried about a dark cloud looming over her future. It wasn't the thunderstorms predicted on Seattle's *Eleven O'clock News*. It was the mere possibility (or maybe probability) of health issues in her not-so-distant future.

She tended to blow off the constant warnings about diet and exercise, making occasional disdainful remarks about how going to the gym was for trophy wives, bodybuilders, and people with way too much time on their hands.

She owned a bakery, after all, and time was limited — especially now as the holidays approached. Somebody had to taste-test the goods for quality assurance.

Judy's generally sedentary lifestyle and steady intake of carbohydrates resulted in a tipping of the scales toward obesity. Yet she was happy and suffered from very few side effects associated with her weight.

"Maybe I'm just meant to be fat and jolly," she joked with one of her employees. "It's got to be good for business — means the pastries are too good to refuse!"

And yet a tiny and very annoying voice in the back of Judy's head constantly reminded her that her health could be in jeopardy. She knew deep down that she was in a high-risk group for diabetes. She was over forty-five, overweight, and diabetes ran in her family.

That night as the TV weather report ended, a health segment on prediabetes began. Judy rolled her eyes and reached for the remote. Then, something made her stop and listen for a few minutes.

Should I be worried? she thought to herself.

* * *

Maybe Judy should talk with her doctor. She has several predictors for insulin resistance (or prediabetes).

What is prediabetes?

Prediabetes is a condition that occurs when blood glucose levels are higher than normal, but they are not yet high enough to be classified as diabetes. The good news is that this condition is often reversible if you take some proactive measures.

The biggest problem with assessing insulin resistance is that it does not have any outward symptoms until you are well on your way to type 2 diabetes. Early detection is very important, and there are some ways in which you can find out if you have prediabetes.

If you find out about insulin resistance early in the game, you have time to make important changes that will stop the progression and possibly avoid diabetes.

Take a short quiz to find out if you are at risk for prediabetes.

Please answer YES or NO to the following questions:

Are you forty-five or older?	YES	NO
Are you overweight or obese?	YES	NO
Do you have high blood pressure?	YES	NO
Do you tend to gain weight around your waist?	YES	NO
Do you eat a lot of carbohydrates?	YES	NO
DO you exercise very little or not at all?	YES	NO
Do you have Polycystic Ovarian Syndrome (PCOS)?	YES	NO
Do you have a relative with type 2 diabetes?	YES	NO
Did you develop gestational diabetes?	YES	NO
Do you have high triglycerides?	YES	NO
Do you have low "good" cholesterol?	YES	NO
Do you have a relative with heart disease?	YES	NO
Have you had a baby who weighed more than nine pounds?	YES	NO
Do you suffer from metabolic syndrome?	YES	NO
Have you ever had an elevated blood glucose test?	YES	NO

If you answered YES to fewer than five of the questions above, it is less likely that you are at risk for prediabetes.

If you answered YES to between five and seven of the questions above, you may be at risk for prediabetes.

If you answered YES to eight or more of the questions above, it is likely that you are at risk for prediabetes.

Lets go over a bit of background information on insulin, glucose, and diabetes in general before getting into symptoms, testing, and treatment for insulin resistance.

Hormones are very important to the regulation of blood sugar in the body. Estrogen, progesterone, DHEA, testosterone, cortisol, and thyroid hormones are all very important in this process.

In women, estrogen will help to lower blood sugar. In men, testosterone lowers blood sugar levels.

Progesterone excess can actually raise blood sugar levels.

Once again, the delicate tapestry of hormones is very important to maintaining a healthy balance in your body, and blood sugar is just one more example of how they are all interconnected.

So, what exactly is insulin?

Insulin is also a hormone, and it is secreted by the pancreas when blood sugar levels rise. Insulin's job is to help glucose (sugar) enter into cells. Once glucose is in a cell, it can be used for energy or stored for future needs.

Insulin binds to cell receptors and provides a pathway for glucose in the blood to move into the cells. It has a pretty important job, as the gatekeeper to let glucose in the door, so glucose can provide the cells with much-needed energy.

What is insulin resistance?

Insulin resistance is when the cells don't respond to the insulin. In other words, insulin's key doesn't work and the door doesn't open. So glucose starts to build up in the bloodstream.

The pancreas senses the glucose in the blood and releases even more insulin. If increased amounts of insulin STILL don't open the cell doors, then you end up with high levels of glucose in your blood. The glucose can't get into the cells, so it has nowhere to go.

Metabolic syndrome was mentioned in the quiz. It is a group of risk factors for heart disease that is connected to insulin resistance. These risk factors include:

- Hyperglycemia (high blood glucose)
- Hypertriglyceridemia (high blood lipids)
- Hyperinsulinemia (high blood insulin)
- Low HDL (low good cholesterol)
- Hypertension (high blood pressure)
- Obesity or overweight
- Waist circumference more than thirty-five inches in women or forty inches in men

You will almost always be prediabetic before developing type 2 diabetes. If you have prediabetes, though, you are not necessarily doomed to end up with diabetes. That is very good news, considering a diagnosis of diabetes means you will be managing your blood sugar levels for the rest of your life.

However, the bad news is that long-term damage may already start to happen when you are prediabetic. The eyes, kidneys, and heart could each be affected by prediabetes.

If you are diagnosed with prediabetes, you can take immediate action to manage your blood sugar levels and prevent or at least delay type 2 diabetes.

What is diabetes?

Diabetes occurs when your body thinks it is in an insulin-deficient state. No matter how much insulin the pancreas generates, the cells in the body do not recognize it, and they do not allow it to open the door for glucose to enter the cells. So, as a result, the cells are deficient in energy from lack of glucose, and the bloodstream has an overabundance of glucose.

Excess glucose in the blood sticks onto proteins in the body, causing dysfunction. This contributes to many serious problems, including blindness, kidney failure, poor wound healing, increased susceptibility to infection, high blood pressure, heart disease, and Alzheimer's, just to name a few.

Excess insulin is also a problem. Insulin is what is called a very *pro-inflammatory* hormone. Inflammation is now recognized as a root cause for many of the chronic diseases associated with aging that you do not want to get, including heart disease, cancer, osteoporosis, autoimmune disorders like multiple sclerosis and rheumatoid arthritis, and dementia.

So the high glucose and high insulin are *both* problematic.

Unfortunately, there are often no symptoms of prediabetes. In fact, the U.S. Department of Health and Human Services has labeled prediabetes as a *silent disease* because there are typically no early symptoms or signs.

If you feel that you are at risk and would like to find out for sure if you have prediabetes, there are a number of tests that may be used to successfully give you a diagnosis.

- **Fasting plasma glucose test**. This is a blood test that measures your glucose (blood sugar) levels after you have gone at least eight hours without eating.

- **Fasting insulin level.** This test measures your insulin level at least eight hours after eating.

- **Oral glucose tolerance test**. This blood test measures your glucose levels after drinking a syrupy glucose-containing drink.

- **Hemoglobin A1c.** This test reflects what your blood sugar levels have been like over the last three months, and does not matter whether you are fasting.

If your blood sugar metabolism is problematic, there are steps you can take to lessen your chances of developing diabetes.

- Cut out sugar! Sugar is a toxin and dramatically increases your risk for diabetes. This includes sugar by any name, including high fructose corn syrup, rice syrup, dextrose, and so on.

- Decrease the trans fat in your diet (found in deep-fried foods and store-bought baked goods such as muffins and crackers — read the labels).

- Reduce the processed starchy carbs in your diet (the white stuff: bread, flour, sugar, rice, potatoes). Even healthier carbs like whole grains, sweet potatoes, and brown rice should be eaten in moderation.

- Eat a diet rich in whole, unprocessed foods such as fruits and non-starchy vegetables (corn and potatoes are the starchiest, so avoid them).

- Exercise regularly. Exercise helps the cells to recognize insulin better.

- Lose weight if you are overweight. The excess fat tissue produces inflammatory chemicals that cause the cells to become more insulin resistant. Losing weight can completely resolve insulin resistance in many cases.

- Taking these steps can dramatically reduce your chances of developing diabetes.

Conclusion

As you now understand, hormones play a very important role in how you feel.

Hormones affect:

- Energy
- Mood
- Sleep
- Memory
- Motivation
- Self-esteem

They are important for the health of your:

- Skin
- Hair
- Heart
- Brain
- Bones
- Muscles
- Urinary tract
- Vaginal lining

Risks for many chronic diseases, including osteoporosis, heart disease, and Alzheimer's, are increased when you are hormonally deficient.

The interplay between your various hormones is complex and is affected by many factors that are in your control. Your nutrition, level of stress, quality of sleep, amount of exercise, and general outlook on life all have an impact. Simply taking hormone replacement without looking after all of these important factors may lead to disappointing results.

The good news is, with some lifestyle changes, you may find that you feel much better very quickly. With the support of a healthcare provider specializing in bioidentical hormone replacement you will be able to regain your sense of vitality and get back to feeling like you again.

Not all women need hormone replacement, and we all have a very unique pattern of hormones. You may need estrogen and progesterone and your next-door neighbor may need thyroid and testosterone. So measuring your hormone levels to learn about your personal pattern is an important first step.

Remember that synthetic hormones are not a match to the hormones your body naturally produces. They are not likely to have exactly the same effects as hormones that ARE an exact match (bioidentical hormones), and some have been shown to have increased risks. If your doctor cannot tell you whether the hormones they are recommending to you are bioidentical or not, then you may want to look for help elsewhere.

Once you have started your treatment, watch for symptoms that may indicate that the dosage is not quite right. Some symptoms of estrogen excess, for example, can include breast tenderness and fluid retention. It could mean that the dose of estrogen was too high for you (we are all very unique and respond differently to the hormones) or it could mean that the balance between estrogen and progesterone is not quite right. A simple dosage adjustment should do the trick and resolve your symptoms quickly. Hormone replacement should help you feel normal again—there should not be any negative symptoms if dosed appropriately.

Once you have been on your treatment for a few months, your hormone levels should be retested. The type of test chosen (saliva, blood, or urine testing) will depend on the form of hormone replacement you are using (topical cream, pills, or pellets, for example). If your doctor is monitoring your levels with blood testing when you are on topical cream, please be aware that the blood test will be underestimating the level of hormones in your tissues and you may be on a dose that is higher than necessary.

But what if your hormones are balanced and you still don't feel your best? Remember that hormone replacement is not a magic pill. You will need to do your part to make sure you are taking care of yourself.

You may also need to consider some other factors that affect your health and the function of the hormones. In fact, some of these issues may have been the cause of the hormone problems in the first place.

Things that you and your doctor may need to consider include:

1. **Hidden food sensitivities.** We estimate that up to one in three women may have an immune reaction to common foods they are eating on a regular basis. While food allergies typically cause symptoms like hives or itching within a few minutes, food sensitivities are different. These are low-grade reactions that happen over several days, so you always have a low level of inflammation that is making you feel tired or bloated or just not your best.

2. **Dysbiosis.** *Dysbiosis* is a new word meaning an imbalance in the microbes living in your intestinal tract. We all have trillions of bacteria and yeast in our digestive tract, and they are incredibly important to our overall health. You may be familiar with probiotics: good bacteria,

often found in fermented or cultured foods like yogurt, that help keep you healthy. Probiotic bacteria keep your colon cells healthy, help you digest your food, make some of your vitamins, regulate your immune system, and do much more. It is common in our modern world to have too much of the wrong bacteria (or even too much yeast, also called *candidiasis*), and not enough of the helpful probiotic bacteria. This can result in bloating, constipation, diarrhea, heartburn, and indigestion. It can also cause problems in other parts of your body as well, including fatigue, brain fog, mood symptoms, joint aches, skin problems, and hormone imbalances.

3. **Environmental toxins.** Many chemicals that we are exposed to on a regular basis act like hormones (but don't show up on our hormone tests). These are endocrine disruptors, mentioned earlier in the book. They can be found in plastics, personal care products like lotions and creams, in pesticide residues, and in materials used in the construction of our homes. A good resource for more information is the environmental working group website (www.ewg.org).

4. **Nutrient insufficiencies.** Even if you are working hard to make sure you are getting your fruits and veggies, the food available to us today does not always contain the maximum amount of vitamins and minerals, due to modern farming practices. If you have hidden food sensitivities, dysbiosis, or environmental toxicities, your digestive lining may not be healthy and you may not be able to appropriately digest and absorb the nutrients in your food. Many of these micronutrients are imperative for normal hormone function.

5. **Unresolved emotional issues.** If you have some major challenges in your life, or past experiences that you have not yet fully dealt with, then simply having balanced hormones may not be enough to help you feel your best. Seeking help for these issues is important.

Too many women have suffered with symptoms, knowing that they don't feel normal. You deserve answers and help getting answers.

Have you had the experience of going to your doctor, explaining your symptoms, having some lab tests done, and then being told that everything is normal?

If everything is normal, then why do you still feel so bad?

Do you feel like your doctor understands that you just don't feel right, but they don't know what to do with you?

Part of the problem is that you and your doctor are looking for different things. You want to feel well; they are making sure you don't have a disease. You would like to figure out what you can do to get better naturally. Your doctor is trained to use drugs and surgery. Unfortunately, most of the time the medicines only put a Band-aid on the symptoms and don't really cure anything. Think about high blood pressure pills, high cholesterol medication, and sleeping pills. What happens if you don't take your medicine? Is the problem really fixed?

Modern medicine has black-and-white thinking: either you have a disease or you don't. But in between, there is a grey area of dysfunction, where you aren't exactly sick, but you aren't well, either.

Hormone imbalances fall in this grey area. But there is help. And you don't have to live with these symptoms. If you are told that you are normal, but you know that you don't feel well, don't give up!

Now that you have been armed with information, you will be able to seek a doctor who can help you get back to being you again.

Best wishes on your journey to wellness.

Appendix

Finding a Healthcare Provider

Ask ten lawyers a question and you will get ten different answers. It is the same with medical professionals. Finding a physician who remembers biochemistry and physiology and who keeps up with new advances is difficult.

Below are listed recommendations of where you can start your search. This approach to your health is simple in theory, but complex to administer. That is why you should look for someone who is willing to spend the time to work with you to sort out the intricacies of your hormonal signature.

Look for a practitioner who uses a functional medicine approach to hormones:

- Replaces hormones as indicated to eliminate or diminish symptoms

- Replaces hormones to the normal physiologic range

- Uses a delivery system that most closely mimics that of the human body

- Replaces deficient hormones with bioidentical hormones only

- Minimizes risks by following the latest medical research findings

- Listens to what patients are saying and partners with them on their journey toward health and vitality

- Monitors with follow-up testing and dose adjustments as required

There are many healthcare providers who can prescribe bioidentical hormones. Find someone with extensive training (more than a weekend course).

You may expect that someone specializing in gynecology would be the best type of practitioner to prescribe hormone replacement. While there are many gynecologists who are expert in the use of bioidentical hormones, most are not. This is not something that was covered in their medical education. You want to look for one who has done extra training and has dedicated their practice to the use of bioidentical hormones.

I recommend looking for a healthcare provider with formal training in bioidentical hormone replacement through an organization such as A4M (American Academy of Anti-Aging Medicine). At the website, www.a4m.com, you can find a list of all their members and you can search by state and country. There are tens of thousands of members, but be sure to ask questions to see if they have competed fellowship training and have passed the written and oral board exams in Anti-Aging and Functional Medicine. If they have completed the fellowship you will see the letters FAARM behind their name (Fellowship in Anti-Aging and Regenerative Medicine). If they have passed the oral exam, you will see the letters ABAARM (American Board of Anti-Aging and Regenerative Medicine).

In order to pass the oral exam, the practitioner must sit in front of experienced doctors and describe in detail how they would care for a patient. They are grilled about all sorts of hypothetical situations and must be highly knowledgeable in order to pass. I have had the privilege of volunteering as a board examiner for many years, and while I may not know the doctor you are considering, I can vouch for the fact that if the doctor has passed this exam, you will know that they possess a reasonable level of competency. This is a voluntary test (it is not required to be able to prescribe bioidentical hormones), and while there are many very good doctors who have not taken the exam, it is a good sign that the doctor has invested a great deal of time and effort in educating themselves to the highest standard in bioidentical hormone replacement.

Another place for doctors to train is the Institute for Functional Medicine. Their website, www.functionalmedicine.org, lists members and whether they have completed a functional medicine training program. If they have passed a voluntary written exam, it will state "IFM Certified Practitioner".

Do a Google search for compounding pharmacies in your community (more about how to find a compounding pharmacy will follow).

Ask your compounding pharmacist; they will know which doctors in the community are prescribing bioidentical hormones and who is doing a good job.

Ask for recommendations from acquaintances who have seen a doctor for bioidentical hormone replacement. If they rave about their doctor, that is a good sign.

Finding a Compounding Pharmacy

Compounding is the practice of individualizing or customizing medications. Pharmaceutical companies mass-produce medications in predetermined dosages. While this meets the needs of most people, there are advantages to individualized dosing, especially in the area of hormone replacement.

Just like not all doctors are experts in prescribing bioidentical hormones, not all compounding pharmacies are expert in preparing bioidentical hormones.

Your doctor can help you find a pharmacy that they trust and work with on a regular basis.

Look for a pharmacy that has PCAB accreditation. This means that they have passed all the requirements to become accredited with the Pharmacy Compounding Accreditation Board. This is not currently a requirement, so you will need to ask the pharmacy if they have voluntarily chosen to demonstrate their high professional standards by participating in this accreditation process. You can search for PCAB pharmacies at www.pcab.org.

The pharmacy should also be affiliated with PCCA (Professional Compounding Centers of America). This is an organization that trains compounding pharmacists to prepare bioidentical hormone prescriptions. You can search for a PCCA pharmacy at www.pccarx.com. Most PCAB-accredited pharmacies will be PCCA members, but most PCCA pharmacies are not yet PCAB accredited.

You can also do an Internet search for compounding pharmacies in your city. If they are PCAB accredited and PCCA members, they should have these proudly listed on their website.

Don't worry! Even if there is no compounding pharmacy near you, most compounding pharmacies will mail your prescriptions directly to your door.

Finding Quality Supplements

Have you been in a store lately, looked at the massive wall of supplement bottles and felt overwhelmed?

It is hard to know where to start.

Unfortunately, there is a lot of variability in the process of manufacturing supplements. Supplements must be of the highest quality (pharmaceutical grade) and free of contamination. While the most expensive supplements are not necessarily the best, cheap supplements are typically cheap for a reason. Your doctor should be able to help you find brands that are high quality and have appropriate doses.

Here are the supplements that I typically recommend to my patients to get them started.

I consider these supplements essential for healthy living:

- **Omega-3 fatty acids:** EPA and DHA (found in fish oil) are the important omega-3 fatty acids that support brain health, eye health, bone health, heart health, blood sugar metabolism, and cancer prevention. They are very anti-inflammatory, so they are important in conditions like arthritis (and any other -itis). They are also important in maintaining healthy hormone balance.

  Don't go by the amount of fish oil in the capsules—the dosage listed on the front of the bottle is often misleading. Go by the amount of EPA and DHA *in* the fish oil. You will need to the look at the total amount of EPA and DHA listed in the ingredient section on the back (you may have to put your reading glasses on for this). If they do not have the amounts of EPA and DHA clearly listed, then it is probably not a very good supplement—they should be bragging about this!

You will also have to take into account how many capsules count as a serving. You want to get at least 1000 mg daily if you are generally healthy. You should be able to get this dose in two capsules, so if your fish oil is not very concentrated, you may want to look for another brand.

- **Vitamin D:** Vitamin D is manufactured in your skin when you are exposed to sunshine. We get very little from our food. People with darker skin need more sun exposure to make adequate Vitamin D.

  If you live farther away from the equator, the sun's rays are less strong, and so more sun exposure is required for adequate vitamin D. If you live in Florida, you will need to spend less time outside than people in North Dakota to get the same amount of vitamin D. But no matter where you live or how fair your skin or how much time you spend outdoors, we are finding that most people need added vitamin D.

  The best place to start is to have your doctor measure your vitamin D level. This has become commonplace; even your regular primary care provider should be willing to do this for you. You may be surprised to learn that your level (like most people's) is low. The lab range varies depending on the lab, and optimally you should be in the upper half of the normal range. Don't be satisfied with your level if it is in the lower end of the normal range. You can start taking D3 (usually between 1000 and 5000 IU daily) and then have your level retested at least three months later to make sure that it has corrected.

- **Pharmaceutical-grade multivitamin:** You already know that you are supposed to eat many servings per day of fresh fruits and vegetables in a variety of colors. According to the food pyramid, depending on your sex and age, it is recommended to have up to ten servings per day. I know that you try, but be honest—when was the last time you consistently achieved ten daily servings of fruits and veggies?

   Most of us do not meet the recommended amounts on a daily basis. Even when we try our best, the foods available to us at the grocery store do not always have the nutrient levels that we would hope for, due to modern farming practices. A multivitamin provides antioxidant vitamins and trace minerals that may help fill any gaps in your diet. It is important to look for a pharmaceutical-grade multivitamin, as many of the common brands contain synthetic forms of the vitamins and poorly absorbable forms of the minerals, limiting their benefit.

You are usually better off buying your supplements from your healthcare provider or from a health food store. Not all the supplements sold at your local grocery store or chain pharmacy are of poor quality, but if I went on a scavenger hunt to find the lowest quality supplements I could find, that is where I would look first. There are many high quality *and* low quality supplements available online, so buyer beware.

Here are some simple things you can look for to check if the supplement you are looking at is a good choice.

- Check the form of Vitamin E. If it says dl-alphatocopherol, that means they have used a synthetic form of vitamin E, which is cheap to manufacture. You wouldn't want to eat synthetic spinach, so why would you want a synthetic vitamin? (Make sure to put your reading glasses on to check this one—the natural form is d-alphatocopherol, which looks very similar.)

- Look at the minerals. Magnesium oxide and calcium carbonate are the less-expensive (and less well absorbed) forms. Examples of minerals that are better absorbed include magnesium citrate and calcium citrate.

- Check the inactive ingredients. There should not be any food coloring. Food coloring is often listed by a Food, Drug, and Cosmetic number; for example, "FD&C#5". No high-quality supplement company would include food coloring. (Do you really care what color your vitamin capsules are?)

- It should not contain sugar. Who hides sugar in a vitamin? Not a high-quality company.

- There should be a list of allergens that are not included in the capsule or tablet. Not every supplement is free of all allergens and fillers, but having a list shows that they are trying to keep out unnecessary ingredients.

Choosing high-quality supplements can be confusing and complicated. Find a doctor who is comfortable using supplements and can recommend good brands.

Next Steps

To schedule an appointment for a hormone evaluation, please give our office a call at 704-752-9346. Let us help guide you on your search for wellness.

Be sure to visit our website at SignatureWellness.org for more information. Sign up for our monthly newsletter to learn more about balancing your hormones.

Like us on Facebook for more information on Health and Wellness.

https://www.facebook.com/Signature-Wellness-235146934865/?fref=ts

About the Author

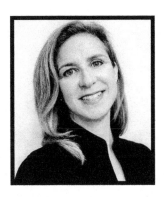

Deborah Matthew, MD, is the founder and medical director of Signature Wellness. Twelve years after graduating from medical school, she decided that she wanted to offer more value to her patients. She knew that emerging science showed that there was more to offer in the areas of preventive medicine and wellness. Dr. Matthew combined her background in medicine with her interest in fitness, health, and nutrition. Her vision is to be able to offer advanced wellness care using scientifically based medical concepts free from pharmaceutical industry bias. This is in response to the observation that despite advances in medicine, preventable illness makes up 70 percent of the health burden in the United States.

Dr. Matthew's area of special focus is in Bioidentical Hormone Replacement. She has completed an advanced fellowship program in Anti-Aging, Functional, and Regenerative Medicine with the American Academy of Anti-Aging Medicine (A4M), passed written and oral exams to become certified in Anti-Aging Medicine, and is currently an A4M Oral Board Examiner. She is a diplomat of the American Board of Integrative Medicine and the American Board of Pediatrics. She is a board member of the North Carolina Integrative Medicine Society and a member of the Institute of Functional Medicine.

Made in the USA
Monee, IL
26 April 2021